Minor Oral Surgery in Dental Practice

Quintessentials of Dental Practice – 27
Oral Surgery and Oral Medicine – 4

Minor Oral Surgery in Dental Practice

By
John G Meechan
Mark Greenwood
Undrell J Moore
Peter J Thomson
Ian M Brook
Keith G Smith

Editor-in-Chief: Nairn H F Wilson
Editor Oral Surgery and Oral Medicine: John G Meechan

Quintessence Publishing Co. Ltd.

London, Berlin, Chicago, Paris, Milan, Barcelona, Istanbul,
São Paulo, Tokyo, New Delhi, Moscow, Prague, Warsaw

British Library Cataloguing-in Publication Data

Meechan, J. G.
Minor oral surgery in dental practice. – (Quintessentials of dental practice; 27.
Oral surgery and oral medicine; 4)
1. Dentistry, Operative
I. Meechan, J. G.
617.6´05

ISBN 1850970823

ISBN 1-85097-082-3

Foreword

Surgery, however minor, carries special responsibilities. These responsibilities include certainty as to the need to operate, having the necessary knowledge and competencies, meeting patient expectations to be skilful and minimally interventive yet effective, and the ability to deal with complications and emergencies as and when they may arise.

Minor Oral Surgery in Dental Practice, volume 27 in the immensely popular *Quintessentials* series, is a modern, authorative and practical consideration of these responsibilities as they relate to surgery in the everyday clinical practice of dentistry. From patient assessment through to managing complications and emergencies, with chapters on surgical principles, relevant pharmacology and the various types of surgery undertaken in clinical practice, the text is logically structured, easy to read, exceptionally well illustrated and peppered with practical guidance – everything expected of a volume in the *Quintessentials* series. In addition, and in common with all the volumes in the series, this book may be read over an evening or two and has been prepared to subsequently make a valuable addition to the reference texts the dental team should have to hand. Overall, this is an excellent addition to the *Quintessentials* series.

Whether you need to update your knowledge and understanding of the surgical aspects of clinical practice, or just wish to reassure yourself that you are up to speed in this regard, *Minor Oral Surgery in Dental Practice* will be a valuable acquisition - an attractive, informative, value-for-money book that will be a pleasure to read and own.

Nairn Wilson
Editor-in-Chief

Acknowledgements

This book could not have been completed without the help of a number of people. Janet Howarth helped with the photography in Newcastle. Figures 7-15 and 7-16 were kindly provided by Mr DG Smith and figures 10-4, 13-1 and 13-6 by Dr Iain MacLeod. Mr RR Patel supplied figures 9-1 and 9-2. Figure 9-10 is a case treated by Mr N Rosenbaum. Figures 5-5b, 5-6, 8-2, 8-6c, 8-12a, 8-12b, 11-3, 11-8a and 11-8b are all reproduced by permission of Oxford University Press from '*Paediatric Dentistry*' , edited by Welbury RR (2001).

Contents

Chapter 1
Introduction

Aim

This chapter describes minor oral surgery and its role in general dental practice.

Outcome

After reading this chapter you should have an understanding of the skills required to successfully practice minor oral surgery.

Surgery in General Dental Practice

General dental practitioners will perform surgical procedures but will not consider themselves to be oral surgeons. What is the scope of minor oral surgery in the general practice setting? A reasonable starting point is the definition that the General Dental Council in the Untited Kingdom used to describe 'surgical dentistry'. This was defined as 'those surgical procedures within the mouth, which would normally be accomplished for a cooperative patient under local anaesthesia with or without sedation in a tolerably short operating time'. These procedures are listed in Table 1-1 and are discussed in this book.

In addition to the skills listed in Table 1-1, the practitioner must be competent in local anaesthetic techniques. The ability to provide safe conscious sedation is also important. These two topics are covered in other books in this series (see reading list).

Medico-legal Considerations

Before embarking on a surgical procedure the dentist should be confident that he or she has the appropriate skills to complete the procedure. If the operation is anticipated to be difficult then the patient should be referred to a more experienced colleague, or to a hospital specialist. Referral halfway through a procedure is not helpful to anyone, especially the patient. If there is any doubt about completing the operation referral is indicated. Indeed it

1

Table 1-1 **Minor oral surgery procedures in general dental practice**

Procedures

- Extraction of teeth and roots
- Management of impacted teeth
- Surgical endodontics
- Exposure of buried teeth
- Excision of benign intra-oral lesions
- Biopsy techniques
- Removal of intra-oral salivary calculi
- Management of dental trauma and oral lacerations
- Management of oro-antral communications
- Dental implantology

may be wise to discuss the option of referral even when the dentist has the appropriate skills. If the patient is informed and offered choices this reduces the chances of litigation. Some patients will prefer the comfort of a familiar face and surroundings when having a surgical procedure. Others may choose to receive such treatment in a specialist centre. Offering the choice does no harm.

The procedure must be properly explained to the patient in order to gain informed consent. This includes a description of the operation, the possible complications, and the post-operative course. It is also important to establish the method of pain control to be used. If this involves general anaesthesia, then this prevents the surgical procedure from being performed in an out-patient surgery in some countries, including the United Kingdom. When conscious sedation is to be used, the patient must be instructed to bring a reliable escort on the day of surgery. This accompanying person is required to take the patient home by car or taxi and ensure that a responsible adult remains with the patient until the next day.

It is important to keep accurate records of the agreed treatment plan and the complications discussed. If the procedure is carried out under local anaesthesia, it is not essential to have written consent. However, this is recommended for surgical procedures. Certainly if the surgery is to be performed under conscious sedation, then written informed consent is essential.

Following surgery, the patient should be given post-operative instructions, preferably in writing. This should include simple first aid measures for control of bleeding and care of the wound. In addition, a contact number for the management of any post-operative emergency should be provided. The clinician should offer advice concerning pain control. If the treatment is carried out under sedation this information is given to the escort.

A review appointment should be arranged. However, the patient should be told to get in touch with the clinician or a designated deputy sooner if there are any concerns.

Conclusions

- Minor oral surgery requires operative and pain control skills.
- Good communication with the patient is important to avoid medico-legal problems.

Further Reading

Craig D, Skelly AM. Practical Conscious Sedation. London: Quintessence, 2004.

Meechan JG. Practical Dental Local Anaesthesia. London: Quintessence, 2002.

Chapter 2
Patient Assessment

Aim

This chapter describes the process of assessing patients who require minor oral surgery, reaching a diagnosis and treatment planning.

Outcome

After reading this chapter you will understand the importance of patient assessment in the practice of minor oral surgery.

Introduction

Comprehensive patient assessment is a prerequisite for successful surgical practice. It is based upon a candid and trusting relationship between patient and clinician.

Competence in the skills of history taking and physical examination is fundamental to this practice. The accurate interpretation of patients' symptoms and the correct eliciting of relevant physical signs provide the basis for diagnosis and treatment planning.

History Taking

Successful history taking involves fascinating detective work. Experienced clinicians can accurately diagnose a patient's problems within the opening minute of a consultation. Only by continued practice and exposure, however, can the less experienced aspire to such intuitive diagnoses. The important principles that facilitate this process comprise:
- introduction
- recording patient details
- the patient's complaint
- history of complaint
- previous medical history
- drug history and allergies
- social history
- case summary.

Introduction

Consultations begin with appropriate social introductions between clinician and patient. A handshake provides not only a polite greeting but also useful information about general health (see later). It must be remembered, however, that a handshake may be inappropriate when dealing with some ethnic groups.

Recording Patient Details

Information regarding the patient's age, sex, racial origin and occupation are extremely important for diagnostic and treatment planning purposes.

The Patient's Complaint

The patient must describe their presenting problem in their own words. The patient's reports of previous clinicians' diagnoses must be regarded with caution. Failure to listen carefully to a patient's history can lead to inaccurate diagnosis and inappropriate treatment.

History of Complaint

The mode of onset of symptoms (sudden or gradual), their time course (constant or intermittent), whether they are worsening, improving or staying the same, and their response to any previous treatment provide invaluable information. The application of this process to the common clinical problem of oro-facial pain is summarised in 2-1.

Previous Medical History

It is often helpful to enquire generally whether the patient has ever been in hospital for any illness or operation, or is currently seeing a doctor for anything. This should take place before asking specifically about a history of heart disease, hypertension, rheumatic fever, breathing problems, diabetes, jaundice, TB, etc. Some important conditions relevant to the practice of minor oral surgery are summarised in Table 2-2 – the medical 'CHALLENGE'.

Drug History and Allergies

It is surprising how often patients fail to appreciate the relevance of medication to surgical practice, prescribed or otherwise. It is therefore best to specifically ask if tablets, pills, medicines, creams, ointments or inhalers of any kind are being used.

Social History

Details of tobacco, alcohol or other recreational drug use must be recorded.

Table 2-1

Oro-facial pain history

1. **SITE** – Point of maximum intensity?

2. **CHARACTER** – Sharp, dull, throbbing, burning?

3. **TIMING** – Date of onset, continuous, intermittent, time of day?

4. **SEVERITY** – How severe, increasing, decreasing, staying the same?

5. **SPREAD** – Where does the pain spread?

6. **RADIATION** – Any other sites affected?

7. **AGGRAVATING FACTORS** – Touch, temperature, pressure?

8. **RELIEVING FACTORS** – Analgesics, heat?

9. **ASSOCIATED SYMPTOMS** – Swelling, discharge, bad taste, dysphagia?

In addition, it is important to determine who will care for the patient following surgery. This is especially important if conscious sedation is being considered.

Case Summary
At the end of history taking, the clinician should:
- recognise all relevant signs and symptoms
- understand the impact of the clinical problem on the patient.
- construct a list of possible diagnoses to aid the clinical examination, which follows.

Patient Examination

Valuable information about patients' general wellbeing can be obtained by careful observation as they first enter the surgery. Their mental state (lucid, cooperative, anxious, depressed), nutritional condition (underweight, over-

Table 2-2

The medical 'CHALLENGE'	
CARDIOVASCULAR DISEASE	– Heart failure Hypertension Ischaemic heart disease Infective endocarditis
HAEMORRHAGIC DISORDERS	– Coagulation defects Platelet disorders
ANAEMIAS	
LIVER DISEASE	– Hepatitis Cirrhosis
LIFE-THREATENING CONDITIONS	– Malignant disease Immunodeficiencies
ENDOCRINE DISEASE	– Diabetes mellitus Thyroid disorders Systemic steroid therapy
NEUROLOGICAL CONDITIONS	– Epilepsy Multiple sclerosis (MS)
GASTRO-INTESTINAL DISORDERS	
RESPIRATORY DISEASE	– Infections Asthma Chronic obstructive pulmonary disease (COPD)

weight or obese), general cardio-respiratory status (pallor, cyanosis, breathlessness, wheeze), the presence of jaundice or skin disease can all be ascertained during these initial moments of consultation. Shaking hands, as introductions occur, can yield additional medical information, such as the metabolic flap of liver disease, finger clubbing, koilonychia, bruising and purpura (Fig 2-1). Detailed and systematic oro-facial examination should be carried out with the patient seated. Appropriate lighting and examination equipment must be available (Table 2-3).

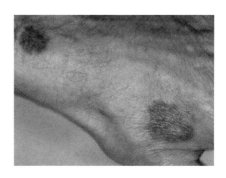

Fig 2-1 Bruising on the hand is suggestive of a bleeding disorder, which should be investigated prior to performing surgery.

Table 2-3

Systematic oro-facial examination	
THE FACE	– Skin colour and complexion Symmetry Bony skeleton Facial nerve function Sensory deficits Eyes
TEMPOROMANDIBULAR JOINTS	– Tenderness Clicks Mandibular movements
MAJOR SALIVARY GLANDS	– Swelling and tenderness Nodular enlargement
LYMPH NODES	– Facial Cervical
LIPS	– Colour Lesions
INTRA-ORAL	– General inspection and salivary flow Buccal mucosa and parotid ducts Tongue dorsum Ventral and lateral tongue Floor of mouth, submandibular ducts and sublingual glands Fauces, tonsils and pharynx Retromolar regions Teeth and periodontal tissues Edentulous ridges Occlusion

Table 2-4

Assessment of an oro-facial swelling

1. ANATOMICAL SITE?

2. SUPERFICIAL or DEEP in origin?

3. SINGLE or MULTIPLE?

4. SHAPE?

5. SIZE?

6. COLOUR?

7. SURFACE – smooth, lobulated, irregular?

8. EDGE – defined, diffuse?

9. CONSISTENCY – fluctuant, soft, firm, rubbery, hard?

10. TENDERNESS or WARMTH on palpation?

11. ASSOCIATED LYMPHADENOPATHY?

An example of the information necessary for assessment of an oro-facial swelling is listed in Table 2-4.

Upon completion of the examination, it is helpful to summarise the salient findings under the term 'special pathology'.

Diagnosis

The diagnostic process requires consideration of the principal mechanisms of surgical disease, as applied to the relevant tissue or organ involved (Table 2-5). This exercise is traditionally referred to as the 'surgical sieve'.

Many diagnoses are apparent after an accurate history and examination have been carried out, although it is sometimes necessary to consider a list of differential diagnoses. Further specialised investigations may be

Table 2-5

Principal mechanisms of surgical disease	
ANATOMICAL ABNORMALITIES	– Congenital Acquired
TRAUMA	
INFLAMMATION	– Acute Chronic
NEOPLASIA	– Benign Malignant
TISSUE GROWTH ABNORMALITIES	– Hyperplasia Hypertrophy Cyst formation
ISCHAEMIA AND INFARCTION	
METABOLIC AND ENDOCRINE DISORDERS	

required to confirm the definitive diagnosis and to aid overall patient management (Table 2-6). Some of these investigations require consultation with other healthcare professionals, such as the patient's general medical practitioner or hospital consultant. It is essential that the clinician determines and records the final, definitive diagnosis before proceeding with treatment planning.

Treatment Planning

A satisfactory treatment plan requires consideration of pre-operative, operative and post-operative care, relevant to the individual patient and their specific disease process. By way of example Table 2-7 summarises the process as applied to the surgical removal of a lone-standing maxillary molar tooth in an elderly diabetic patient on anticoagulant medication.

Table 2-6 **Further investigation for minor oral surgery**

Further investigation	
ORO-FACIAL	– Tooth vitality tests Local anaesthetic injections Oral microbiology swab Fine needle aspiration biopsy (FNAB) Tissue biopsy
GENERAL	– Temperature Pulse Blood pressure Respiratory rate Weight Electrocardiogram (ECG)
HAEMATOLOGY and BIOCHEMISTRY	– Full blood count Clotting studies Urea and electrolytes Blood glucose Liver function tests Serum calcium
RADIOLOGY	– Dental panoramic tomograph (DPT) Periapical views Occlusal views

As mentioned in Chapter 1, it is often appropriate for the practitioner to refer the patient for treatment elsewhere. The reasons for referral include:
- surgical competence
- need for general anaesthesia
- underlying medical condition.

Many patients who require surgical dentistry and who suffer from medical conditions can be treated in a general dental practice. As a rough guide the use of the American Society of Anesthesiologists (ASA) classification of medical fitness is helpful (Table 2-8). This system provides a numerical value to patient health. Patients who are classified as ASA III or above are best treated in specialist centres.

Table 2-7

Treatment planning example

CASE HISTORY — Elderly non-insulin dependent diabetic patient on warfarin (post-pulmonary embolus) requiring extraction of a lone-standing maxillary molar.

PRE-OPERATIVE — GENERAL PREPARATIONS
Ensure use of all regular medications and normal diet
Out-patient local anaesthetic appointment with accompanying person
Up to date INR blood test (consider warfarin adjustment in consultation with patient's physician if INR >4.0)
Consider use of pre-emptive analgesia and prophylactic antibiotics (but beware interactions between aspirin, NSAIDs and metronidazole with warfarin)

DENTO-ALVEOLAR — Radiographic assessment
Informed patient consent
Specific warnings re: tuberosity fracture, oro-antral communication (OAC)

OPERATIVE CONSIDERATIONS — Local anaesthetic administration
Transalveolar surgical approach
Identification and management of any surgical complication.

POST-OPERATIVE CARE — Regular analgesic medication
Possible need for antibiotics or ephedrine nasal drops if OAC created.
Importance of maintaining normal diet
Written post-operative instructions and contact telephone number for advice
Care at home upon discharge

No matter where the patient is treated, part of the treatment planning process includes consultation with other healthcare workers involved in the management of medically compromised patients. It is better to receive advice that might prevent potential problems in advance rather than seek help to manage an acute complication or emergency (see Chapter 14).

Table 2-8

ASA fitness scale	
ASA I	Normal healthy patients
ASA II	Patients with mild systemic disease
ASA III	Patients with severe systemic disease that is limiting but not incapacitating
ASA IV	Patients with incapacitating disease that is a constant threat to life
ASA V	Patients not expected to live more than 24 hours

Conclusions

- Thorough assessment of the patient is essential for the safe practice of minor oral surgery.
- The taking of a good history is important in obtaining an accurate diagnosis.
- The patient's medical status impacts on the practice of minor oral surgery.

Further Reading

Moore UJ (ed). Principles of Oral and Maxillofacial Surgery. 5th edn. Oxford: Blackwell Science, 2001.

Scully C, Cawson RA. Medical Problems in Dentistry. 5th edn. Oxford: Wright, 2004.

Chapter 3
Principles of Minor Oral Surgery

Aim

This chapter describes the principles involved in minor oral surgery.

Outcome

After reading this chapter you should have an understanding of the principles involved in the successful practice of minor oral surgery.

Introduction

As mentioned in Chapter 2, the successful practice of any form of surgery begins by taking a thorough history, reaching the correct diagnosis and formulating an appropriate treatment plan. Arriving at a diagnosis may involve performing pre-operative special tests such as radiography and pulp testing. Treatment planning includes the choice of anaesthesia.

It is imperative that the surgeon has a thorough knowledge of the anatomy of the area of interest. Surgery should be aseptic and as atraumatic as possible. The operator must have the appropriate instrumentation. Suggested instruments are listed in Table 3-1 and shown in Fig 3-1.

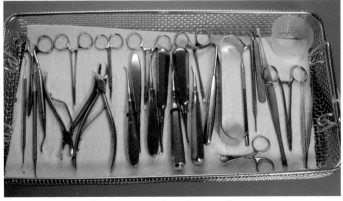

Fig 3-1 A tray of instruments for minor oral surgery.

Table 3-1

Suggested instrumentation for minor oral surgery
Scalpel handle and blades (11 and 15)
Periosteal elevators (Howarth's)
Tissue retractors (Bowdler Henry/cheek/tongue)
Surgical handpiece and burrs
20ml syringes for irrigation
Bone files
Rongeurs
Chisels
Osteotomes
Curettes (Mitchell's trimmer)
Artery clips (Mosquito)
Scissors
Tissue forceps
Suture holders and sutures (resorbable and non-resorbable)
Dental elevators (straight (Couplands) and curved (Warwick James/Cryers))
Dental extraction forceps
Mirror
Dental probe

It is worth considering the steps involved in the removal of a buried root as an aid to discussing the principles. These steps are:

• gaining informed consent
• localisation of the root
• operative pain control
• incision
• flap design
• flap raising
• bone removal
• root removal
• curettage and debridement
• wound closure
• post-operative pain control
• review.

Gaining Informed Consent
This was discussed in Chapter 1. When performing surgical procedures it is good practice to obtain written consent. Written informed consent is essential when conscious sedation is used.

Localisation of the Root

This is achieved by clinical examination, both visual and by palpation. In addition radiographs are needed. Radiographs are useful because they:

- aid in localisation
- show any associated pathology
- indicate the quality of surrounding bone
- demonstrate the proximity of important structures.

Occasionally, it may be necessary to take different radiographs to locate the root using parallax. Such views may be two different intra-oral periapical films or panoramic and occlusal views.

Operative Pain Control

It is imperative that pain control is excellent if surgery is to be performed. As mentioned in Chapter 1, the mainstay for minor oral surgery is local anaesthesia with or without sedation. If pain control is unsatisfactory the procedure cannot be performed to the best standards. Excellent local anaesthesia has benefits at both ends of the syringe. The patient feels no pain and the clinician can work with reduced stress. The use of sedation can be helpful for some patients. However, sedation must not be used as a measure to counter poor local anaesthesia. This topic is discussed further in Chapter 4.

Incision

The incision should be made with a sharp disposable blade. If a number of incisions are involved the blade should be changed. The blade normally used in intra-oral surgery is the number 15 (Fig 3-2). A number 11 blade may be used on occasion (Fig 3-2).

The scalpel handle should be held like a pen and the incision made at 90° to the surface. When making an incision for a mucoperiosteal flap the incision

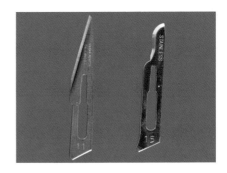

Fig 3-2 Scalpel blades numbers 11 (left) and 15 (right).

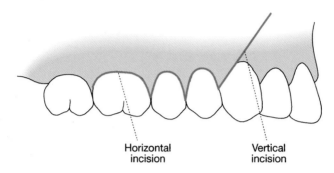

Fig 3-3 A flap design with vertical and horizontal incisions.

is made down on to bone. This is important, as it means that when the flap is raised the bone is directly exposed and there is no soft tissue attached. Pressing the scalpel on to bone during the incision can blunt the blade. This is why the blade should be changed when there are multiple incisions.

Flap Design
The design is such that the flap:
- is mucoperiosteal
- has an adequate blood supply
- avoids damage to important structures
- allows adequate visibility
- allows atraumatic reflection
- has its edges on sound bone at the end of the procedure
- can be replaced at the end of surgery without tension.

Many flaps have vertical and horizontal incisions (Fig 3-3). The vertical incision is made in such a way that the base of the flap is wider than the free-edge – this is to ensure an adequate blood supply. The vertical incision should not split interdental papillae. The vertical incision is located in a position that avoids important structures such as the mental nerve. In addition the vertical incision should be placed in such a position as to ensure it is over sound bone at the end of surgery.

The horizontal incision is normally a gingival margin incision. It should be long enough to ensure adequate visibility with atraumatic reflection. Wounds heal across the incision rather than along the cut, therefore long

18

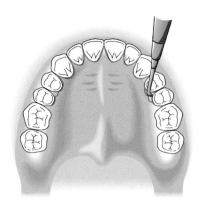

Fig 3-4 A Warwick James elevator being used to begin flap raising.

incisions heal as quickly as short ones. Thus keeping incisions too small offers no advantage. Indeed, small flaps can be damaged if they are retracted with force to afford visibility. This may delay healing. The various flap designs used are described in the relevant chapters later in this book.

Flap Raising

It is important when raising a mucoperiosteal flap to avoid damaging the periosteum. Damage can occur at two stages of raising the flap. First, the periosteum may be torn if the elevator is improperly positioned. This is avoided by ensuring that the incision is down to bone and that the elevator is inserted in the plane between bone and periosteum. The use of a curved Warwick James elevator (Figs 3-4 and 5-4) to begin flap raising before resorting to a periosteal elevator can help in this regard. Secondly, the periosteum may be perforated during the act of raising from bone. This is avoided by ensuring that the curve of the elevator is pointing towards bone and not towards the soft tissues (Fig 3-5).

Bone Removal

Bone is removed for the following reasons:
- to expose the buried root or tooth
- to improve access and visibility
- to relieve bony impaction
- to create space for elevators or forceps
- to create a fulcrum for elevators
- to reduce dead space at the end of surgery.

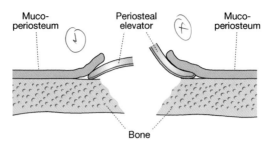

Fig 3-5 When using a periosteal elevator the curve should point to the bone (left) not to the soft tissues (right) as this can perforate the flap.

Bone can be removed by a number of methods including:
- handpiece and burs
- chisels and osteotomes
- rongeurs
- bone files.

Handpiece and burs
When using a bur a straight surgical handpiece is used. The normal speed is 40,000rpm. The bur that is most commonly used is a round number 8 surgical bur. Alternatively a fissure bur can be employed. Copious irrigation with sterile saline is important. An air rotor should not be used as this can force air under the flap, leading to surgical emphysema.

Bone can be removed by two techniques when a bur is used. The bone can be removed piecemeal or 'en bloc'. One way of achieving the latter is the 'postage stamp' method. This involves outlining the area of bone to be removed with a series of perforations (Fig 3-6). These are then connected and then the entire piece of bone removed. Alternatively the area can be outlined as a continuous cut and then removed.

Chisels and osteotomes
Chisels may be used by hand pressure or with a mallet. The use of a mallet is not recommended in the conscious patient. Hand pressure is effective in removing bone in young patients. In older patients it is only useful in the maxillary buccal bone. Chisels have a chamfer and a straight edge (Fig 3-7). The chamfer should be placed next to the bone that is being removed, as this part of the instrument produces the most damage. Osteotomes differ from chisels in that they have chamfers on both aspects of the working edge (Fig 3-7). They are used to split bone or teeth when using a mallet.

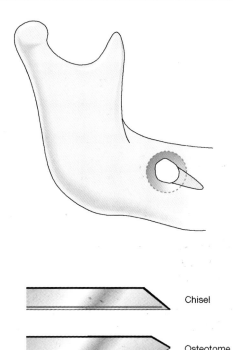

Fig 3-6 The postage stamp method of bone removal.

Fig 3-7 A chisel (top) has a single chamfer, an osteotome (below) has a double chamfer.

Chisel

Osteotome

Rongeurs
Rongeurs are also known as 'bone-nibblers'. They are available in two forms known as end-cutting and side-cutting. These differ in the position of the working edge. They are useful in removing interdental and inter-radicular bone and reducing the sharp edges of socket walls.

Bone files
Bone files can be used to reduce sharp pieces of bone at the end of surgery. They are available as pull and push designs that differ in the orientation of the 'teeth' at the working end (Fig 3-8).

Root Removal
Once the root has been exposed it can be removed by forceps or elevators, as described in Chapter 5.

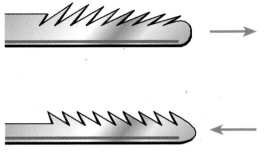

Fig 3-8 Bone files are either used with a pushing (top) or a pulling (below) motion.

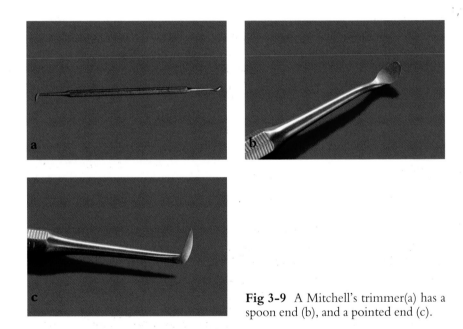

Fig 3-9 A Mitchell's trimmer(a) has a spoon end (b), and a pointed end (c).

Curettage and Debridement

It is important to remove loose pieces of bone and root together with any soft-tissue pathology at the end of the procedure. An important area to inspect is between the raised periosteum and the bone. This is achieved by thorough irrigation with sterile saline and instrumentation. The spoon end of a Mitchell's trimmer is useful in this regard (Fig 3-9). Any abnormal soft

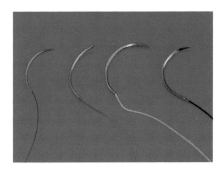

Fig 3-10 Sutures used in minor oral surgery. From left to right: 6/0 nylon, 4/0 vicryl, 3/0 vicryl rapide and a 3/ 0 black silk.

tissue removed should be sent for histological examination in a specimen pot containing 10% neutral buffered formalin (see Chapter 13).

Wound Closure

The wound should be closed with sutures (Fig 3-10). Sutures are classified by their circumference and design of needle. The larger the number the narrower is the suture. The suture chosen should be weaker than the tissue being operated upon. In the mouth the 3/0 type is ideal for closing wounds in attached and reflected mucosa. A curved cutting needle is recommended. Clinicians will determine which length and curvature of needle suits them best. Resorbable varieties such as vicryl are suitable for most intra-oral wounds. Non-resorbable monofilament sutures such as nylon are used on the superficial layer of skin wounds. They can also be used intra-orally. On facial skin fine sutures (5/0 or 6/0) are used. When resorbable sutures are used to close the deeper layers of facial wounds an undyed variety should be chosen.

When using sutures to close wounds in the mouth the needle should be inserted at 90° to the surface. The point of insertion is about 3mm from the wound edge (Fig 3-11a). When closing the surface layer of a skin wound it is best to evert the wound edges. To achieve this the 'bite' taken at the deep surface is wider than that taken superficially (Fig 13-11b).

Simple interrupted, mattress or continuous sutures may be used to close mucosal wounds (Fig 3-12). When deep wounds are being closed the layer immediately below the surface should have the knots buried (Fig 3-13). This technique may be used with resorbable sutures for the superficial layer intra-orally to decrease discomfort by eliminating bulky knots, which may irritate the tongue or lips.

When non-resorbable sutures are used intra-orally, they should be removed

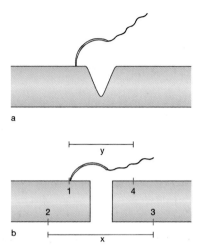

Fig 3-11 (a) The needle is inserted at 90° to the surface of mucosal wounds. (b) To evert skin wounds a larger bite is taken at the deeper surface (the dimension 'x' is longer than 'y').

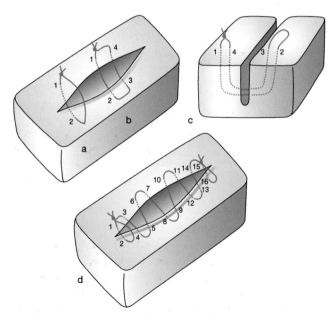

Fig 3-12 Different sutures: (a) Single interrupted. (b) Horizontal mattress. (c) Vertical mattress. (d) Continuous.

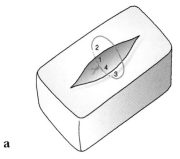
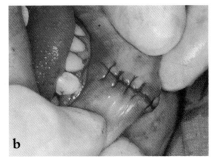

Fig 3-13 A buried knot. (a) The technique. (b) Clinical appearance.

between five and seven days post-operatively. On skin they should be removed at five days.

Post-Operative Pain Control

The patient should be given advice concerning post-operative pain control. This is discussed in Chapter 4.

Review

The patient should be reviewed about one week post-operatively to ensure that healing is progressing satisfactorily.

Principles of Management of Infection

The practitioner performing minor oral surgery must have an understanding of the principles relating to the management of infection. These are:

- removal of the cause
- institution of drainage
- prevention of spread
- restoration of function.

The most important of these principles and the only curative procedure is removal of the cause. The other measures are supportive. Thus it is important to remove the cause at some stage. The sooner the cause is removed the better. This can eliminate the need for antibiotic therapy. This benefits the patient and is important in a global sense, as it may help limit the number of resistant organisms. Removing the cause may also institute drainage and will prevent spread.

When removal of the cause does not create drainage, then this must be achieved by other means. This usually means incision at the most dependent part of the swelling. A drain may have to be inserted to keep the pathway open. Rubber drains or parts of rubber dams can be used to achieve this.

Sometimes the management of infection merits referral to a specialist maxillofacial unit. This is certainly the case if there is any danger to the airway. Urgent referral is important if there is evidence of swelling in the floor of the mouth, as this can rapidly lead to airway obstruction. Other indicators for referral are the need for intravenous antibiotics and fluid replacement.

Conclusions

- Successful surgery relies on good history taking, diagnosis and treatment planning.
- The dentist performing minor oral surgery must have a sound knowledge of relevant anatomy.
- A number of general principles apply to minor oral surgery procedures.
- The most important principle in the management of infection is removal of the cause.

Further Reading

Pedlar J, Frame J. Oral and Maxillofacial Surgery. Edinburgh: Churchill Livingstone, 2001.

Wray D, Stenhouse D, Lee D, Clark A. Textbook of General and Oral Surgery. Edinburgh: Churchill Livingstone, 2003.

Chapter 4
Pharmacology and Minor Oral Surgery

Aim

This chapter describes the use of drugs in minor oral surgery.

Outcome

After reading this chapter you will have an understanding of the use of drugs to aid the practice of minor oral surgery.

Introduction

The successful practice of surgery is dependent upon the proper use of drugs. The most obvious example is the provision of anaesthesia during surgical procedures. This chapter will consider the following:

- pain control
- anxiety control
- antibacterial drug use
- other agents used in minor oral surgery.

Pain Control

Pain control is important at two stages of surgery. These are:

- operative pain control
- post-operative pain control.

Operative Pain Control

The practice of pain control for minor oral surgery involves the use of local anaesthesia with or without conscious sedation (see below). The need for general anaesthesia requires referral to a specialist centre such as a hospital clinic.

What is the best local anaesthetic for surgical dentistry? A number of factors have to be considered. An important one is the patient's medical status. On the basis that the patient is healthy, what is the best choice? In order to reduce operative haemorrhage, a vasoconstrictor-containing solution is required (Fig 4-1). Two different vasoconstrictors are available in local anaesthetic

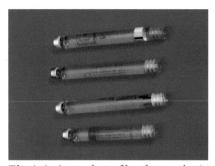

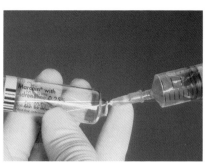

Fig 4-1 A number of local anaesthetic solutions are available for use in dental cartridges. A vasoconstrictor containing solution such as lidocaine with epinephrine is the local anaesthetic of choice for surgical procedures in the mouth.

Fig 4-2 Long acting local anaesthetic solutions such as bupivacaine or levobupivacaine can aid post-operative pain control.

solutions in many countries. These are epinephrine (adrenaline) and felypressin (octapressin). The former produces superior haemorrhage control. Thus an epinephrine-containing solution is preferred.

The use of long-acting local anaesthetics such as bupivacaine or levobupivacaine may help in reducing post-operative pain (see below). However, the operative anaesthesia they produce is not as good as lidocaine with epinephrine. Additionally, in some countries the long-acting agents are not available in dental local anaesthetic cartridges (Fig 4-2).

Therefore the solution of choice is 2% lidocaine with epinephrine. Mepivacaine (2%) with epinephrine or 4% articaine with epinephrine are alternatives although the latter is best avoided if block anaesthesia is being used, given the potential problem of long-lasting paraesthesia with this drug concentration.

Post-operative pain control
As mentioned above, the use of long-acting local anaesthetics such as levobupivacaine can prolong the duration of anaesthesia and thus reduce post-operative pain experience. It is important to point out that, to achieve this effect, long-acting agents must be employed as regional blocks. When used as infiltration anaesthesia there may be prolonged soft-tissue numbness, but the onset of post-operative pain does not differ from that occurring after the use of a conventional local anaesthetic such as lidocaine.

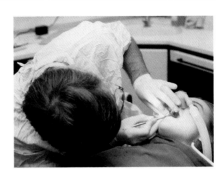

Fig 4-3 Inhalation sedation is a useful aid when providing minor oral surgery in children.

The mainstay of post-operative pain control is the use of analgesics. As the pain of surgery is inflammatory in nature, it is best controlled by non-steroidal anti-inflammatory drugs. When non-steroidals are contraindicated the drug of choice is paracetamol (up to 1g four times daily). The pain usually begins in the early post-operative period and thus the early use of analgesics is essential. Indeed, the ideal time to commence analgesic therapy is before surgery begins. This is because non-steroidal analgesics prevent the occurrence of pain rather than treat an established pain. The use of analgesics prior to surgery is known as pre-emptive analgesia. Surprisingly, studies into the effectiveness of pre-emptive analgesia have shown conflicting results. Ibuprofen and COX 2 inhibitors have shown a pre-emptive effect. COX 2 inhibitors are not recommended at present, as they have been implicated in the production of cardiovascular complications. Thus the drug of choice is ibuprofen, unless contraindicated. When using ibuprofen a dose of 400mg should be taken around 30 minutes before surgery. Therapy should continue for a variable time dependent upon the surgery performed. The pain following soft tissue biopsy reduces considerably within 24 hours. On the other hand, discomfort following the removal of third molar teeth is still apparent at the third post-operative day. Thus, patients who have third molars removed should be advised to continue taking analgesia for at least three days after surgery (e.g. 400mg of ibuprofen three times daily).

Anxiety Control

The use of conscious sedation can be helpful in the provision of minor oral surgery. In young patients the use of inhalation sedation (relative analgesia) can allow surgical procedures to be performed (Fig 4-3). The only area where problems arise is when operating in the maxillary anterior region - for example, when performing a midline fraenectomy (see Chapters 8 and 9). This is because the nasal mask interferes with surgical access.

Intravenous conscious sedation with midazolam (or propofol) permits the performance of surgery in adult patients. Midazolam allows about 45 minutes operating time, which is the period of pulpal pain relief afforded by conventional dental local anaesthetics. In addition the use of midazolam affords pharmacological protection against the CNS toxicity effects of lidocaine, so it is useful when larger doses of local anaesthesia are being used.

Antibacterial Drug Use

Antibiotics are used in minor oral surgery for two purposes. These are:
- therapeutic use
- prophylactic use.

Both of these will be discussed.

Therapeutic use

Antibacterial drugs are used to treat bacterial infections. They have a supportive role in the treatment of dental infections. They are not curative. Thus they should only be used to control an infection that is not immediately amenable to surgical treatment. This means they have a limited role to play in the management of dental infections, most of which are readily treated by surgical intervention. As stressed in Chapter 3, the only cure for an infection is the removal of the cause. Antibiotic therapy does not achieve this in dental infections.

Situations where an infection may need to be controlled include those where access to the surgical site is not possible - for example, due to trismus. If trismus is associated with swallowing or breathing difficulties, immediate referral to hospital for extraoral drainage under general anaesthesia is essential. Over 90% of the bacteria responsible for infections of dental origin (excluding periodontal infection) are susceptible to the following antibacterial drugs:
- penicillins
- metronidazole
- erythromycin
- clindamycin.

These are the drugs that should be considered to treat dental infections. The best method is to take a sample of the infection. This may be either pus or a swab. This should be cultured for identification and sensitivity. This is not always practicable. Thus, prescribing is often empirical. The first choice is a broad-spectrum penicillin such as amoxicillin. A loading dose of 3g may be administered orally; the typical maintenance dose is 250mg three times daily. Metronidazole (200–400mg three times daily) is used for anaerobic infections, which can often be suspected by their characteristic smell. Erythromicin (250mg four times daily) is used in those allergic to penicillin. Clindamycin (150–300mg four times daily) has a reputation for producing pseudomembranous ulcerative colitis. In order to avoid this serious complication this drug should not be used for long periods.

The duration of antibacterial therapy should be until clinical resolution occurs. There is no point in continuing drug therapy once this has been achieved. 'Completing the course' after resolution offers no advantage but increases the chance of producing resistant organisms.

Prophylactic use
The prophylactic use of antibacterial drugs can be classified into two categories:
• prevention of wound infection
• prevention of distant infection.

Antibacterial drugs that are used prophylactically must be bactericidal.

Prevention of wound infection
Wound infection is uncommon after minor oral surgery. This is due to the excellent blood supply in to the mouth in most patients. Thus the site of surgery does not inherently increase the incidence of infection. Factors that increase the chances of wound infection are:
• long procedures
• transplantation/implantation
• decreased host resistance.

Long procedures are those that exceed two hours of operating. This should not occur in minor oral surgery in dental practice.

Transplantation and implantation procedures should be performed under antibacterial prophylaxis.

Decreased host resistance may be encountered in the practice of minor oral surgery. Decreased host resistance may be localised or systemic. An example of a localised decrease in resistance to infection is the mandible irradiated as part of therapy for malignant disease (Fig 4-4). Systemic decrease in

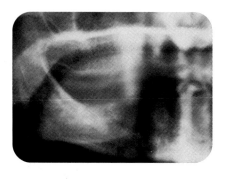

Fig 4-4 An area of necrosis in the right mandible due to decreased resistance as a result of therapeutic irradiation to treat an oral malignancy.

resistance might be due to illness or immunosuppressant therapy. When host resistance is reduced then prophylactic use of antibacterial drugs is indicated. When using antibacterial drugs to prevent infection it is important that the correct timing of administration is chosen. The object is to obtain maximum levels of antibacterial agent in the blood clot. It is not possible for the drug to enter the clot three hours after formation. Thus the drug must be administered prophylactically with the aim of achieving optimum concentration at the end of the procedure. Thus when using a drug such as amoxicillin it should be administered orally one hour before the end of the procedure. A dose of 3g is given. Alternatively it could be given as a 1g dose intravenously during the operation. As the antibacterial agent cannot enter the clot three hours after formation there is no point in giving the patient a prescription to pick up the drug after surgery.

Prevention of distant infection
Procedures that breach the tooth/periodontal tissue junction run a risk of producing an endocarditis in 'at-risk' patients. Surgical procedures involving the teeth are in this category. The timing of antibacterial therapy in these cases is different to that mentioned above. Therapy is aimed at producing optimum plasma levels of the antibacterial agent at the start of the procedure. Thus, if oral amoxicillin is being used, it should be taken one hour before the procedure begins. Recommended regimens for the prophylaxis of endocarditis are regularly updated and practitioners are advised to consult appropriate national publications such as the *British National Formulary*.

Other Agents Used in Minor Oral Surgery
A number of other agents may be used in minor oral surgery. These include prophylactic corticosteroids, antiseptic mouthwashes, antifibrinolytic agents and nasal decongestants.

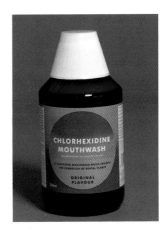

Fig 4-5 Antiseptic mouthwashes can be useful before and after intra-oral surgery.

Some surgeons advocate the use of prophylactic corticosteroids to reduce the incidence of post-operative problems. The evidence for the efficacy of such regimens in minor oral surgery is inconclusive. Findings from studies investigating the use of oral steroids pre-operatively are not convincing. Intravenous dosing can provide short-lived improvements in swelling, trismus and post-operative pain.

Antiseptic mouth rinses can be used before and after intra-oral surgery to maintain oral hygiene (Fig 4-5). Patients should be advised that some agents such as chlorhexidine-containing rinses can cause staining of the teeth, but that this can readily be removed. Such rinsing is best avoided immediately after surgery, as it can precipitate haemorrhage. It is better to begin gentle rinsing the day after surgery.

Antifibrinolytic agents such as tranexamic acid mouthwash can be useful aids in the management of patients with bleeding disorders. As mentioned in Chapter 14, patients with significant bleeding problems, such as haemophilia, should be managed in the hospital environment.

Nasal decongestants may be prescribed to patients who have had surgery involving the maxillary antrum (see Chapter 10). When using drugs such as ephedrine, it is important to ensure that therapy is not prolonged. When used for more than two weeks, ephedrine can cause a rebound vasodilation, which can exacerbate antral problems.

Concurrent Drug Therapy

It must be remembered that the practice of surgery may be influenced by drug therapy the patient is receiving. This applies to both prescribed and non-prescribed agents, including the use of illicit drugs. Many drugs interfere with haemostasis, typically by reducing the number of platelets. Other drugs may interfere with wound healing. As mentioned in Chapter 2, it is imperative to take a thorough drug history from surgical patients as therapy may necessitate referral, or the use of appropriate prophylaxis.

Conclusions

- The successful practice of surgery depends upon the use of appropriate drug therapy.
- The taking of a drug history is important prior to the performance of minor oral surgery.

Further Reading

Meechan JG, Seymour RA. Drug Dictionary for Dentistry. Oxford: Oxford University Press, 2002.

Seymour RA, Meechan JG, Yates MS. Pharmacology and Dental Therapeutics. Oxford: Oxford University Press, 1999.

Chapter 5
Extraction of Teeth and Roots

Aim

This chapter aims to describe the techniques and instruments that can be employed in order to extract teeth and roots.

Outcome

After reading this chapter you should understand the principles of tooth and root removal.

Introduction

The extraction of teeth is a commonly performed operation that can be a simple task. It may however rely on a high degree of skill to be accomplished successfully in all cases. Success depends on understanding both the morphology of teeth, or more exactly their roots, and the anatomy of the supporting tissues and associated structures, together with the vascular and nerve supply. Careless technique can create problems for future replacement of missing teeth (chapter 9). Advances in dental care and a more elderly population have resulted in patients maintaining teeth until the elastic qualities of their support are all but exhausted. This creates special management problems for the performance of minor oral surgery.

In this chapter the basics of tooth extraction will be explored, although it is likely that most dentists will already have skills in this area.

Tooth Morphology

The following aspects of tooth morphology are important:
• number of roots
• shape of roots
• diversity of form
• proximity to important structures.

It is essential to be familiar with the morphology of the teeth to better understand the way in which forces applied to them will achieve their removal. In addition, it is essential to appreciate the diversity of the morphology in certain teeth. This is particularly the case with third molars and upper premolars. Finally, the proximity of roots of teeth to vital structures such as the inferior alveolar nerve and the maxillary antrum should always be remembered to avoid inadvertent iatrogenic damage.

Forceps

The following aspects of extraction forceps are important:
- the design of the beaks
- the fit to root surfaces
- the handles should give ergonomic grip
- the efficient delivery of force.

The ideal way to apply force to a tooth would be with 'steel fingers'. This would allow the ultimate proprioceptive feedback from the site of the extraction to the clinician. Forceps should be considered as the next best thing. They are designed to achieve the delivery of force to the tooth in the most ergonomic way possible. There are a number of different designs (Fig 5-1). For example, there are differences between those forceps designed for the removal of permanent teeth and those used to extract deciduous teeth (Fig 5-2). In addition, when removing adult lower molar teeth two distinct patterns of beak are available. In the standard lower molar forceps there are two pointed beaks that engage the roots in the bifurcation area. Force is then applied in a buccal direction to deliver the tooth (see below). In the cowhorn design the pointed beaks are designed to slide below the furcation and deliver the tooth in a vertical direction as the forceps beaks approximate (Fig 5-3a). Such deeply plunging beaks should not be used on deciduous teeth as they may damage the underlying permanent tooth, and smaller deciduous lower molar forceps should be employed (Fig 5-3b). Practitioners will develop particular choices for any given situation. In general forceps apply forces to the tooth, which in turn expands the alveolar bone and ruptures the periodontal ligament to allow removal.

Elevators

Dental elevators are often used in extractions. They:
- apply force directly to tooth
- are used by rotation

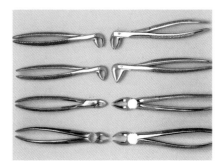

Fig 5-1 The various designs of dental extraction forceps. Those designed for the deciduous dentition are shown on the left, those for permanent teeth on the right.

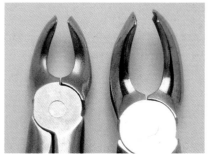

Fig 5-2 A comparison of the size of beaks in upper deciduous molar (left) and upper permanent molar (right) forceps.

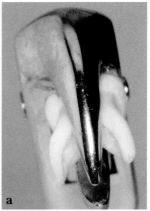

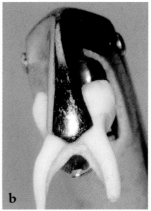

Fig 5-3 (a) The cowhorn design should not be used on deciduous teeth as damage to the underlying permanent successor could occur. (b) When removing deciduous lower molar teeth lower deciduous molar forceps are recommended.

- are used to facilitate forceps extraction
- engage dentine with their working edge.

Elevators differ from forceps in that they apply force directly to the tooth to lift it out of its socket. An understanding of the different ways in which force can be applied to teeth allows greater subtlety to be used in achieving success in extractions. Elevators are available in several designs, the most popular of which are the Couplands, Warwick James and Cryers (Fig 5-4).

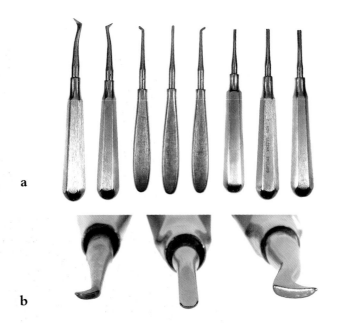

Fig 5-4 (a) The different designs of dental elevators. From left to right: two Cryers, three Warwick James and three Couplands. (b) details of a curved Warwick James (left), a Couplands (centre) and a Cryers (right).

Although they seem radically different they are all based on a working edge and a curved cross-section. All elevators should be used by rotation, similar to a screwdriver when used to insert or remove a screw. This harnesses the ratio between the width of the blade and the handle to employ the principle of secondary leverage. Elevators should never be used as primary levers as the forces generated may cause damage to adjacent teeth or simply break the tooth to be extracted.

Couplands elevators can be used both as direct elevators and as dilators of the socket. This is down to the design of the instrument, which is similar in shape to a single beak of a pair of forceps (Fig 5-5a). The blade of the Couplands can be advanced along the periodontal ligament to expand the buccal or palatal bone in order to reduce the resistance of the tooth to movement (Fig 5-5b). This is particularly useful in the upper jaw where the buccal alveolar bone is thinner than that in the mandible.

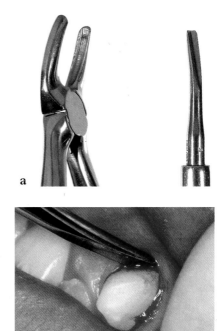

Fig 5-5 (a) The Couplands elevator is equivalent to one beak in a pair of forceps. (b) A Couplands elevator being wedged between the alveolar bone and tooth to expand the socket.

Radiographs

As mentioned in Chapter 3, pre-operative radiographs are an invaluable aid to assessment prior to tooth extraction and should show:

- condition of crown
- angulation of tooth
- root abnormalities
- bone density
- periodontal condition
- adjacent teeth and roots
- position of important structures.

A periapical radiograph may show this information but a panoramic view such as the dental pantomograph (DPT) can provide a wider view of the surgical problem.

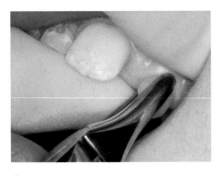

Fig 5-6 The fingers and thumb of the supporting hand are in close proximity to the tooth being extracted.

Tooth Extraction

An extraction involves the following stages:
- exploration of the path of movement
- use of combination of instruments
- use of two specific forces
- vertical force toward apex
- buccal movement or rotation.

The extraction of a tooth should be a process of exploration of the way in which the tooth will most easily move. This is then exploited by the use of various instruments. Both forceps and elevators are employed by experienced clinicians to ascertain the most efficient route to success. Even the testing of local analgesia by probing the periodontal ligament may give useful information concerning bone density and level. This helps gauge the resistance of the tooth to movement.

Force is used in two quite specific ways. Firstly, a force must be applied along the long axis of the tooth towards the apex. This ensures that the forceps are advanced as far apically as possible. Whilst maintaining this apical force a second force is employed concurrently to move the tooth either in the bucco-palatal/lingual direction, or to rotate it. Multi-rooted teeth are usually delivered in a buccal direction, as lingual or palatal movement of the forceps is limited by the other jaw. Single-rooted teeth with round root cross-sections, such as upper incisors or lower premolars, can be rotated and then withdrawn vertically. For these forces to be successful in removing rather than fracturing a tooth, the clinician must develop an awareness of what is happening to the tooth. This is appreciated through the finger and thumb grip of the forceps and the fingers of the supporting hand, which should be as close as possible to the site of the extraction (Fig 5-6).

Once the tooth is removed the socket walls are compressed by finger pressure to return them to their original position. The patient is not discharged until bleeding has ceased. Normally the socket fills with a healthy blood clot within a few minutes of completion of the extraction. If bleeding continues then pressure is applied. This is achieved by the patient biting on sterile gauze placed over the socket. If haemorrhage continues then the steps outlined in Chapter 14 are followed.

Surgical Extraction

The principles underlying surgical extraction were explained in Chapter 3. Surgical extractions consist of the following steps:
- bone exposure by raising a mucoperiosteal flap
- root exposure by removal of alveolar bone
- division of roots as indicated
- delivery of tooth with elevators or forceps.

Surgical extraction may be essential when difficulty is encountered during the extraction of a tooth or when root fracture occurs. It should be considered a logical extension of the extraction technique. The abstract nature of the problem encountered is exposed to direct vision. The improved access gained by raising a mucoperiosteal flap, together with bone removal, should allow a successful outcome of the procedure without unduly increasing its morbidity.

A mucoperiosteal flap should be designed to give adequate access without compromising vital structures such as the mental nerve. The principles of flap design were outlined in Chapter 3. Designs usually incorporate a gingival margin incision, cutting the gingival attachment, coupled with a relieving incision through the periosteum to give flexibility of the tissue. The design should ensure edges of the wound lie on sound bone and incising through frenae should be avoided as scarring can be more marked. The incision should be made with a sharp blade held to ensure the mucosa is cut at right angles to its surface and the incision should be carried through the complete depth of soft tissue to bone. Particular attention should be paid to incising around the gingival papillae to avoid undue force, and thus trauma, when lifting them from the bone. This should enable the mucoperiosteal flap to be raised as a 'sandwich', with the only damage to the soft tissue occurring at the point of the incision.

The flap should be dissected from underlying bone using sharp instruments to facilitate the raising of the periosteum. Bone should be exposed cleanly.

Once raised, the flap is retracted to protect it and allow the clinician to remove bone safely. This is achieved using a handpiece and sharp bone burs with a sterile irrigation system. Suction should be employed by the assistant to allow the clinician unhindered vision. Bone removal continues until adequate exposure of the root has been achieved. This is difficult to estimate exactly but, in general, in multi-rooted teeth the bifurcation should be clearly exposed to ensure accurate division where necessary. Great care must be taken when removing bone close to the mental or inferior alveolar nerves to protect these structures from damage by the burs.

The roots of the tooth may be elevated, or forceps applied if the crown is intact to deliver the tooth. Debridment and wound closure follow removal as described in chapter 3.

Complications

Major complications of extractions are uncommon. Most problems are readily addressed at the time. The complications of minor oral surgery are discussed in Chapter 14.

Conclusions

- Successful extractions rely on the proper application of force.
- Successful extractions require proper instrumentation.
- Surgical extractions are sometimes required to successfully remove teeth.

Further Reading

Moore UJ (ed). Principles of Oral and Maxillofacial Surgery. 5th edn. Oxford: Blackwell Science, 2001.

Chapter 6

Management of Impacted Teeth

Aim

To discuss the assessment and describe the surgical management of impacted teeth.

Outcome

After reading this chapter, you should have an understanding of the assessment of impacted teeth, and how such teeth should be managed.

Impacted Teeth

Impacted teeth are frequently found during routine clinical and radiographic examination. Once discovered, the clinician has to decide whether or not the tooth should be removed. Once the decision to remove the tooth has been made, the method of anaesthesia and surgical technique should be selected. This has to be done with an appreciation of the potential surgical complications.

What is an Impacted Tooth?
Impaction occurs when there is prevention of complete eruption into a normal functional position within the dental arch, caused by obstruction by another tooth, or development of the tooth in an abnormal position.

Which Teeth Become Impacted?
The tooth most commonly impacted is the mandibular third molar, with the maxillary canine the second most frequently impacted tooth with a prevalence of 1.7%.

Assessment of Impacted Teeth
Once an impacted tooth has been discovered, its position relative to the surrounding structures needs be assessed. This is usually done radiographically (Fig 6-1). Once the position of the tooth has been established, the clinician has to decide what to do about it.

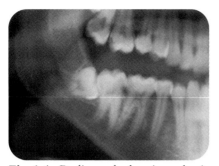

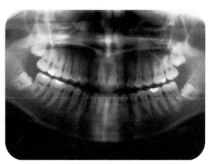

Fig 6-1 Radiograph showing a horizontally impacted right mandibular wisdom tooth. The roots are lying close to the inferior alveolar nerve canal which can be clearly seen.

Fig 6-2 A dental panoramic radiograph showing four unerupted and impacted third molar teeth. The roots of both mandibular third molars are in close proximity to their respective inferior alveolar nerve canals.

The decision to remove a symptomatic tooth is usually straightforward. This is guided by the need to relieve the patient's symptoms, such as pain or infection. The difficulty arises with asymptomatic impacted teeth found during routine clinical examination or, more frequently, by radiographic examination (Fig 6-2).

There are a number of treatment options. The tooth can be left alone with periodic assessment; it can be surgically removed, or surgically exposed to encourage spontaneous eruption or facilitate orthodontic alignment. A further option of tooth transplantation may also be considered in certain circumstances (see Chapter 8).

Foremost in the decision-making process should be the wish of the patient, who must make the final decision. This judgment will normally be based on guidance given by the clinician. This should include indications for and against any proposed treatment. The different options are described below.

Observation of an Impacted Tooth
Doing nothing is a decision that often finds great favour with the patient. Although there may be no indication to remove the impacted tooth at that point in time, the patient should be made aware of any potential future complications that the impacted tooth may cause, when left untreated. Tooth movement, resorption of adjacent teeth and cyst formation are the main risks (Figs 6-3 and 6-4).

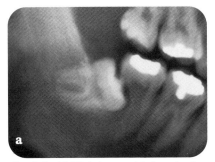
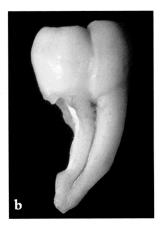

Fig 6-3 (a) This lower third molar has caused extensive resorption of the root of the adjacent second molar. (b) The degree of resorption can easily be seen on the extracted second molar.

An impacted tooth that does not warrant treatment should be monitored periodically by both clinical and radiographic examination. This is to detect any change in position or a developing local pathology.

Surgical Removal of the Impacted Tooth

There are a number of indications for the surgical removal of an impacted tooth. Clinical guidelines such as those produced by the UK National Institute for Clinical Excellence (NICE) are useful in this regard. The indications for surgery are described overleaf.

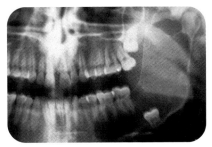
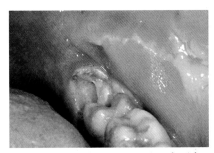

Fig 6-4 A cyst associated with the crown of the unerupted left mandibular third molar, that has expanded to involve a large part of the mandible including the coronoid and condylar processes.

Fig 6-5 Pericoronitis associated with a partially erupted left mandibular wisdom tooth.

45

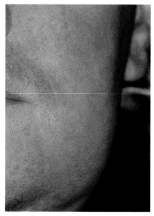

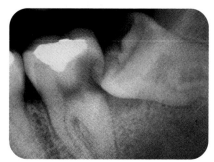

Fig 6-6 Cellulitis associated with an impacted left mandibular wisdom tooth.

Fig 6-7 Caries in the distal aspect of the second molar due to the impacted third molar.

Infection

When there is a history of infection, in particular recurrent infection, this is usually localised - such as pericoronitis, which is the commonest reason for the removal of impacted third molars (Fig 6-5). Cellulitis or abscess formation can also occur in relation to impacted teeth (Fig 6-6).

Caries

The impacted tooth should be removed when it is carious, or when it is the cause of caries in an adjacent tooth (Fig 6-7).

Pulpal or Periodontal Pathology

The presence of pulpal and/or periapical pathology is an indication for removal of an impacted tooth.

Periodontal disease, in particular when associated with an adjacent tooth, can often be arrested by removing the impacted tooth.

Resorption

When an impacted tooth has developed internal or external resorption, or there is resorption of an adjacent tooth (Fig 6-3), it should be removed. This

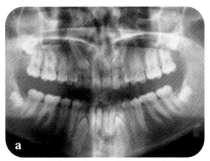 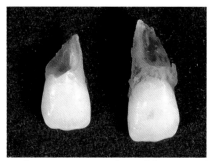

Fig 6-8 (a) Both maxillary canines have caused extensive resorption of the roots of the permanent lateral incisor teeth. (b) The extracted lateral incisor teeth showing extensive root resorption.

can be a major problem in adolescent patients, in whom root resorption of the incisor teeth can be expected in about 12.5% of incisors adjacent to an ectopic canine (Figs 6-8 to 6-9).

Other Pathology

Impacted teeth should be removed if they are the cause of, or are associated with, pathology. Examples include disease of the follicle associated with the crown of an unerupted impacted tooth. This may be a cyst or tumour.

When an impacted tooth is lying in the line of a fracture it may be removed if it interferes with fracture reduction. This is often the case with impacted mandibular third molar teeth (Fig 6-10).

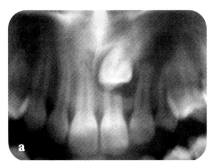 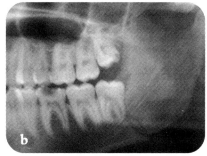

Fig 6-9 Even the roots of central incisor teeth may be resorbed by ectopic canine teeth.

Fig 6-10 A fracture of the mandible passing through the socket of the unerupted third molar.

To Aid other Treatment

Removal of an impacted tooth may be indicated to allow:
- the orthodontic alignment of the adjacent teeth
- orthognathic or reconstructive surgery of the jaws. Impacted mandibular third molars are often removed around nine months prior to a sagittal splint mandibular osteotomy to facilitate surgery and reduce morbidity
- restorative treatments such as the placement of a fixed prosthesis or dental implants.

Medical Factors

When the patient has a specific medical condition, such as endocardial or valvular heart disease predisposing them to bacterial endocarditis, the prophylactic removal of an impacted tooth is often indicated to eliminate the potential risk. There may also be an indication to remove impacted teeth for patients with organ transplants. The same applies to patients who are to undergo chemotherapy or receive radiotherapy to the jaws.

Maintenance of the Impacted Tooth

There are occasions when impacted teeth should not be removed. For example, there is usually no indication to surgically remove an impacted tooth that is completely covered with bone and which does not meet any of the above indications for surgery.

Very occasionally, despite reasonable indications to remove an impacted tooth, it may be left *in situ* due to a potential risk, such as permanent damage to the inferior alveolar nerve, which might outweigh any possible benefit to the patient.

Surgical Exposure
This procedure is often carried out prior to orthodontic alignment, which is usually necessary to 'disimpact' the tooth. Surgical exposure alone is unlikely to lead to spontaneous alignment. The patient should therefore be willing to wear fixed orthodontic appliances (Fig 6-11). Exposure may be open or closed. Open exposure involves soft-tissue sacrifice. In closed exposure, the tooth is surgically exposed, an orthodontic appliance attached, and the flap replaced. This is discussed in Chapter 8.

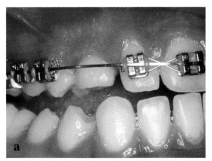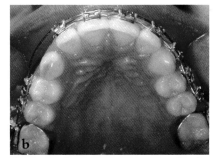

Fig 6-11 (a) This patient has a fixed orthodontic appliance to create space for the unerupted canine tooth. The deciduous canine is still in situ. (b) An occlusal view showing the space created within the arch to accommodate the permanent canine, prior to transplant.

Surgical Transplantation

Surgical transplantation of an unerupted and impacted tooth is an option for the patient who is unwilling to undergo orthodontic alignment and is seeking a quick-fix treatment. The alternative is tooth removal and prosthetic replacement.

Transplantation should only be considered when conditions permit; there should be sufficient room within the dental aches to accommodate the tooth, both between the adjacent teeth (Fig 6-11b), and within the occlusion. This is discussed in Chapter 8.

Surgical Management of Impacted Teeth

Anaesthesia

Local anaesthesia, either alone or supplemented by conscious sedation, is appropriate for the removal of many impacted teeth. When surgical access is expected to be difficult - for example, in palatally impacted maxillary canines - general anaesthesia may be more appropriate. General anaesthetic is usually required for the surgical removal of unerupted impacted teeth in children.

Surgical Removal of the Impacted Tooth

There are generally five stages to removing an impacted tooth. These are:
- raising the mucoperiosteal flap
- bone removal

- sectioning the tooth
- debridement
- wound closure.

The principles behind these stages were described in Chapter 3.

Raising the Mucoperiosteal Flap
There are several designs of flap that may be utilised, but they all follow the same basic principles. Relieving incisions, if used, should lie on sound bone at the end of the procedure; the flap should therefore extend at least one full dental unit in front and one unit behind the impacted tooth.

Examples of flap designs are shown in Fig 6-12. Design of the flap should take account of important anatomical structures such as the mental nerve, and be modified accordingly.

When raising a mucoperiosteal flap to remove an impacted mandibular wisdom tooth, there should be no reflection of the lingual soft tissues in order to avoid injury to the lingual nerve.

Bone Removal
Following reflection of the mucoperiosteal flap, bone is removed using a surgical drill fitted with a round surgical bur. Copious irrigation with sterile saline is important to reduce morbidity. It is important not to use an air turbine handpiece as air can be forced under the soft issues. This may lead to surgical emphysema. This is a surgical emergency if it results in airway obstruction.

Great care must be taken to avoid damage to the roots of the adjacent teeth, which are often in very close proximity to the impacted tooth. Care must also be taken to avoid injury to the inferior alveolar and lingual nerves, which may be very near to the impacted tooth (Fig 6-13).

Sectioning the Tooth
Once the impacted tooth has been sufficiently exposed, it may be possible to remove it whole. Alternatively it can readily be sectioned with a fissure bur on a surgical handpiece, and removed in pieces.

Debridement
Once the tooth has been successfully removed, it is important to irrigate the socket with sterile saline to remove any surgical debris and bone fragments.

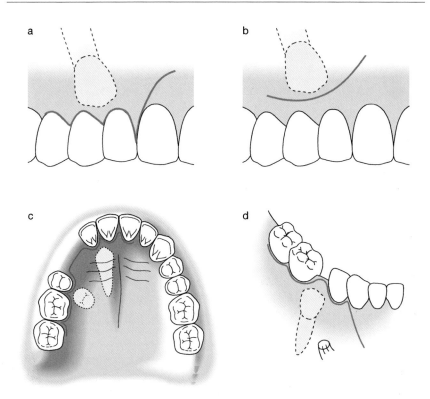

Fig 6-12 Diagram showing different designs of mucoperiosteal flap. (a) A buccal flap for the removal of an unerupted maxillary canine tooth that is lying buccal to the adjacent teeth. (b) If the tooth is lying quite high, then an incision can be made in the sulcus, but the incision should be at least 5mm above the attached gingiva. (c) For an unerupted maxillary canine or second premolar tooth that is palatally displaced, a palatal flap should be raised. (d) A buccal flap for an impacted mandibular second premolar tooth. The anterior relieving incision should be placed far enough anteriorly to avoid damage to the mental nerve.

Fig 6-13 The right mandibular wisdom tooth has been surgically removed. A lingual mucoperiosteal flap was raised, and in the process the lingual periosteum was torn. The lingual nerve can be clearly seen adjacent to the socket, showing how close and vulnerable it is to injury during third molar removal.

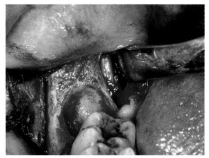

Any sharp bony edges must be smoothed with a surgical bur or with bone files; otherwise they may cause pain and discomfort or even breakdown of the overlying mucosa. Any pathological soft tissue associated with the impacted tooth should also be carefully removed. The spoon end of a Mitchell's trimmer is useful in this regard. If there is any doubt as to the nature of the material removed it should be sent for histological examination, as described in Chapter 13.

Wound Closure

The mucoperiosteal flap is then repositioned and carefully sutured into position using resorbable sutures, such as 3/0 vicryl. The number of sutures used should be sufficient to retain the flap in its original position but without undue tension. Usually the gingival margin incision is approximated using sutures passed through the interdental spaces. The vertical incision is closed with single interrupted sutures, although sutures are not always necessary in this region. The patient is not discharged until post-operative haemostasis is achieved.

Surgical Removal of Impacted Mandibular Third Molars

A buccal mucoperiosteal flap is raised to expose the impacted third molar tooth. An incision of 1–1.5cm is made backwards from the distal aspect of the second molar along the external oblique ridge of the mandible; incisions of greater length than this risk injury to the long buccal nerve. The incision is then extended forwards and downwards into the buccal sulcus (Fig 6-14). Retraction of this flap gives good access to the buccal aspect of the third molar.

Bone is then removed with an irrigated bur to expose the tooth. No bone should be removed from the distal aspect of the tooth as there is a risk that the bur may perforate the lingual plate and damage the lingual nerve. The greatest risk of this happening is during the removal of distoangularly impacted third molars. Once sufficient buccal bone has been removed, the tooth can be sectioned and removed in pieces. Again great care must be taken during tooth sectioning to avoid drilling all the way through the tooth as this can also lead to damage to the lingual nerve.

Once the tooth has been removed, the bony margins of the socket should be smoothed as described above, and the socket irrigated with copious amounts of sterile saline solution. The mucoperiosteal flap is replaced and sutured in position.

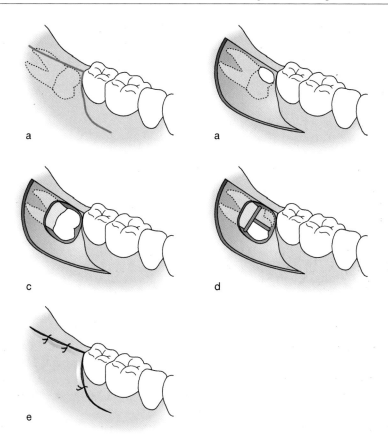

Fig 6-14 Surgical removal of mandibular third molar teeth. (a) An incision is made down the external oblique ridge of the mandible to the back of the second molar and then extended down into the sulcus. (b) The muco-periosteal flap is revealed and reflected. The mucosa above the tooth is then elevated and freed, but only to the internal ridge of bone. No lingual flap is raised. (c) Bone is removed on the buccal aspect only to expose the crown of the tooth. (d) The tooth is then sectioned, using a bur, and elevated in pieces. Great care is required to ensure that the bur does not penetrate the lingual bone while drilling. (e) After the tooth has been removed the bone edges are smoothed, the socket is copiously irrigated and the flap secured back in position with sutures.

This common oral surgical procedure is associated with a high incidence of short-term morbidity; pain, swelling and trismus. Of more concern are the potential long-term complications of injury to the inferior alveolar and lingual nerves, which can result in numbness of the patient's lower lip and tongue. About 4% of patients sustain an injury to their inferior alveolar nerve during removal of their lower third molars, but there is little evidence that this incidence is dependent upon the surgical technique used.

The incidence of injury of the lingual nerve is approximately 7%, and the surgical technique employed for surgery does affect the incidence of damage to this nerve.

The standard surgical technique used for the removal of impacted mandibular third molars involves the elevation of a buccal mucoperiosteal flap. Some practitioners, primarily in the UK, were taught to elevate the soft tissues overlying the tooth and alveolar crest distal to the tooth, and then place a periosteal elevator between the lingual periosteum and the lingual plate of bone. The purpose of this last procedure is to displace all of the soft tissues on the lingual side, including the lingual nerve, away from the third molar, thus protecting the nerve during bone removal and tooth-sectioning. The retraction of a lingual flap in this manner is associated with an increased incidence of damage to the lingual nerve, and there is good evidence that it should be avoided in most cases.

Maxillary Third Molar Teeth

There are few indications to remove unerupted maxillary third molar teeth. Upper third molars that are in the line of proposed orthognathic surgery are often removed at the same time as the lower third molar teeth for the same reason. Occasionally, mesioangularly impacted third molars can give rise to pain and are removed.

An incision is made along the alveolar crest distal to the second molar and then extended forwards and upwards into the upper buccal sulcus (Fig 6-15). Elevation of the mucoperiosteal flap affords very good access to the third molar, which can often then be elevated without any bone removal. Where necessary, a small amount of buccal bone is removed with either an irrigated bur or chisel. Following irrigation the flap is replaced, and secured with sutures (Fig 6-15).

Maxillary Canine Teeth

Maxillary canine teeth normally develop and erupt on the buccal aspect of the dental arch. A buccally positioned canine tooth will occasionally become impacted, usually as a consequence of loss of space within the arch. Such

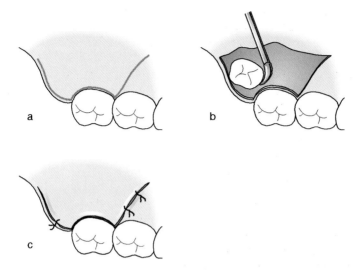

Fig 6-15 Surgical removal of unerupted maxillary third molar teeth. (a) An incision is made across the tuberosity to the back of the second molar, then up into the sulcus. (b) Once exposed, the upper third molar can often be elevated without the need to remove bone. (c) Following debridement and copious irrigation, the flap is secured with sutures.

teeth can be readily removed, if such treatment is indicated, by raising a buccal mucoperiosteal flap and elevating the impacted tooth (Fig 6-12a).

Maxillary canine teeth that develop on the palatal aspect of the dental arch frequently become impacted and fail to erupt. Surgical removal of these teeth can be difficult, and careful pre-operative assessment of their position is essential. Unless the tooth is deemed to be lying just beneath the palatal mucosa a general anaesthetic may be the preferred option, in particular in the younger patient.

An incision is made in the gingival crevice on the palatal aspect of the maxillary teeth, extending from the second premolar to the midline (Fig 6-16). A palatal mucoperiosteal flap is then raised, reflecting the mucosa away from the teeth to expose the canine area. Considerable force may be needed to raise the flap as the palatal mucosa is firmly bound to the underlying bone. Bone is removed using either an irrigated bur or chisel before the canine is elevated. The bone margins are smoothed, and following debridement the flap is sutured in place using interproximal sutures.

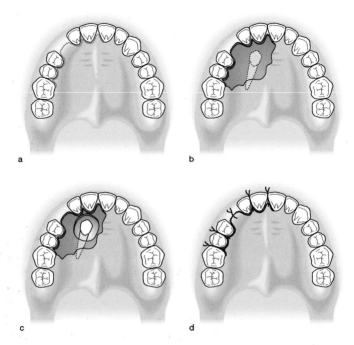

Fig 6-16 Surgical removal of impacted canine teeth. (a) An incision is made in the gingival crevice. (b) A muco-periosteal flap is raised and retracted. (c) Bone is removed using an irrigated bur or chisel to expose the canine tooth, which can then be elevated. (d) The flap is repositioned and held in place with sutures.

Perioperative Medication

Surgery to remove or expose impacted teeth will invariably lead to pain and discomfort, but the degree and intensity of pain can vary greatly. The removal of an unerupted and impacted tooth that has remained asymptomatic, will often lead to surprisingly little post-operative discomfort. The removal of an impacted partially erupted mandibular third molar can, however, cause the patient to suffer quite severe post-operative pain. The clinician should therefore recommend post-operative analgesics appropriately, as described in Chapter 4.

The clinician should also make the patient aware of the post-operative pain-time cycle. Following third molar removal, the patient will not experience the greatest level of pain when the local anaesthesia wears off, but five to seven hours after surgery. As described in Chapter 4, analgesic intake is best begun prior to surgery.

The prescribing of antimicrobial agents is not usually indicated following surgery to expose or remove impacted teeth. Nevertheless, many clinicians do prescribe antimicrobials after third molar surgery. The administration of steroids, either pre- or perioperatively is also used by some to reduce the degree of post-operative swelling and discomfort. This was discussed in Chapter 4.

Complications

Complications following surgery to remove impacted teeth are rare. Post-operative pain, swelling and trismus can be expected. Post-operative haemorrhage may be a problem, but in most cases can be arrested with firm pressure applied by the patient biting on a gauze swab. When this is not sufficient the haemostatic procedures outlined in Chapter 14 should be performed. Persistent bleeding after these measures suggests that the patient may have an underlying bleeding problem, which the pre-operative assessment failed to detect. In such cases the patient should be referred for haematological investigation. Post-operative infections are not common and can usually be treated with the antibiotics described in Chapter 4.

The main long-term complication following the surgical removal of teeth is nerve damage as described above. It is therefore very important, when obtaining informed consent, to make patients aware of the possibility of nerve injury prior to their surgery, including the possibility, albeit small, of permanent sensory loss.

Conclusions

- Teeth frequently are impacted.
- Some impacted teeth remain symptomless.
- Some impacted teeth will produce symptoms necessitating their removal.
- Each impacted tooth should be fully assessed prior to surgery.
- The specific possibility of nerve injury should be assessed.
- The patient must be made aware of the possible risks involved, including the possibility of permanent nerve damage during third molar surgery.

Further Reading

National Clinical Guidelines. London: Faculty of Dental Surgery of England, 1997.

Robinson PP, Loescher AR, Yates JM, Smith KG. Current management of damage to the inferior alveolar and lingual nerves as a result of removal of third molars. Br J Oral Maxillofac Surg 2004;42:285-292.

Chapter 7

Surgical Endodontics

Aim

This chapter will describe the indications for, contraindications to and techniques of surgical endodontics.

Outcome

After reading this chapter you should know when surgical endodontics should be performed and the surgical techniques to be employed.

Introduction

The term surgical endodontics encompasses a number of procedures. This chapter will consider the following:

- apicectomy
- repair of a lateral perforation
- root resection.

Apicectomy

Apicectomy means removing the apical portion of the root of a tooth. It is performed to remove atypical or complex apical foramina, together with abnormal, typically infected adjacent tissue.

It is important to establish at the outset that apicectomy is not an alternative to effective conventional endodontics. A simple explanation as to why apicectomy is inferior to good quality endodontics is that it is never performed under rubber dam. Other reasons include:

- decreasing the crown:root ratio (Fig 7-1)
- exposing accessory canals at the apex (Fig 7-1)
- increasing the area of root filling material exposed at the apex (Fig 7-1)
- iatrogenic damage to important structures (Fig 7-2).

Advances in endodontics, including the use of microscopes, have resulted in a reducing need for endodontic surgery. This is progress, as apicectomy is not an ideal treatment for a compromised tooth. The only thing worse is extraction,

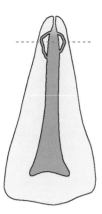

Fig 7-1 Removing the apex of a tooth can expose accessory canals and increase the area of root filling exposed.

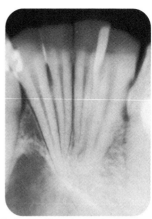

Fig 7-2 Performing apical surgery on one of these lower incisors could easily damage one of its neighbours.

and this at least more or less guarantees a cure. Thus, apicectomy should be considered the last stop before the terminus of extraction. Not only is apicectomy a poor alternative to good conventional endodontics, it should not be considered if the existing root filling is less than ideal. Apicectomy should not be performed on a tooth with inadequate coronal restorations. This is because any coronal leakage will result in the failure of apical surgery. When bony support for the tooth is poor - for example, as a result of periodontal disease - surgery may worsen the support. Thus it is difficult to argue the case for surgical endodontics. In addition, if the patient's general health is poor, surgery is contraindicated unless essential. Thus the contraindications to apicectomy are:

- unsatisfactory endodontics
- coronal leakage
- poor bony support
- where support will be insufficient following surgery
- poor periodontal health
- poor general health.

Notwithstanding the above, surgical endodontics is still performed. So there are times when this procedure is indicated. The indications for apicectomy are:

- when it is impossible to clean, shape and fill root canals to within 1–2mm of their apical extension with conventional endodontics
  - fractured instrument
  - severe dilacerations
  - immovable post (of a well-fitting crown) (Fig 7-3)

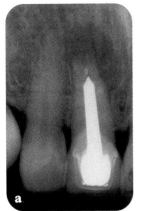 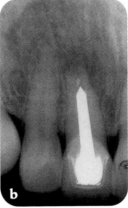 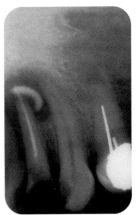

Fig 7-3 (a) A tooth with a well fitting crown with an apical area. (b) The area has healed following apical surgery.

Fig 7-4 Excess root filling material at the apex of a tooth associated with apical infection. Apical surgery is indicated to remove this material.

- when excess root canal material or a broken instrument is present through the apex and is giving rise to problems (Fig 7-4)
- to remove a fractured apical portion
- external root resorption (Fig 7-5)
- when an apical biopsy is required.

Radiographic Assessment

It is essential to have good radiographs before performing apical surgery. A long-cone paralleling technique periapical film showing at least 3mm of tissue beyond the apex of the appropriate tooth is ideal. If a large apical radiolucency is associated, then a sectional panoramic radiograph should also be taken.

Technique

The technique must allow:
- access to the apex of the tooth
- good visibility of the apex of the tooth
- good healing.

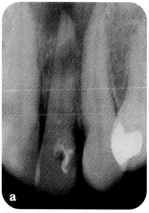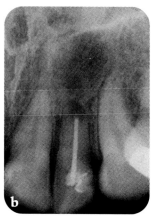

Fig 7-5 (a) Periapical pathology associated with external root resorption of an upper lateral incisor. (b) healing after apicectomy.

Description of the technique is divided into:
- anaesthesia
- flap design
- bone removal
- apicectomy
- curettage
- apical seal
- wound closure

The procedure is illustrated in Fig 7-6.

Anaesthesia
Apical surgery is well suited to local anaesthesia. A combination of regional block and infiltration should suffice. The infraorbital nerve block in combination with infiltrations is particularly useful when dealing with upper anterior teeth. Good anaesthesia should be established before raising the flap. Once a flap is raised ooze of the anaesthetic solution can reduce efficacy and tastes awful.

Flap Design
A number of different flaps have been advocated for apical surgery (Fig 7-7). These can be described as:
- those involving the gingival margin
  - two-sided (Figs 7-6a, b and 7-7a)
  - three-sided (Fig 7-7b)

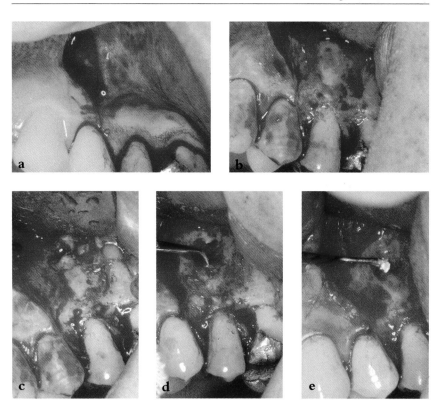

Fig 7-6 (a) Flap for apicectomy of upper second premolar showing vertical and horizontal incisions. (b) Flap raised to reveal bony defect at apex of upper second premolar. (c) Apicectomy of tooth revealing root canal. (d) Preparation of root canal for retrograde filling with ultrasonic tip. (e) Filling of retrograde cavity with IRM. (f) Wound closure.

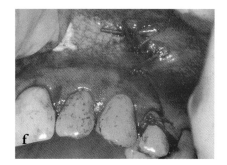

- those not involving the gingival margin
  - semi-lunar (Fig 7-7c)   – vertical (Fig 7-7e)
  - horizontal (Fig 7-7d)   – Luebke-Oschenbein (Fig 7-7f)

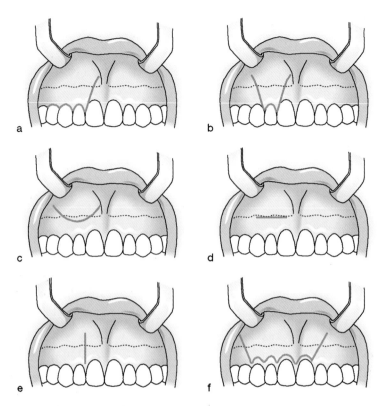

Fig 7-7 The different designs of flap used for apicectomy.

The two- and three-sided flaps have the potential to disrupt the gingival position on the tooth being treated. However, these flaps do allow excellent access to the apex of the tooth and are helpful in orientation. This is particularly useful when treating malaligned teeth. Semi-lunar and horizontal flaps do not directly interfere with the gingival margin but can make orientation difficult. In addition, it is all too easy for part of the wound to end up over a bony defect at the completion of the procedure. This is common when the amount of bony destruction is greater than predicted pre-operatively. This can lead to wound breakdown. The vertical flap has the advantage that sutures are not always required at the end of the surgery. This flap provides limited access, however, and is more difficult to retract.

Bone Removal
Bone removal should be performed with a surgical handpiece and burs under

copious irrigation with sterile saline. A balance has to be made between provision of sufficient access to the apex while being as conservative as possible to the alveolus and the root. When there is a defect in the buccal bone the decision as to where to start drilling is easy. The defect is the place to commence bone removal. This should continue in a radial manner until the apex is located. When no defect is obvious a useful tip is to use a sharp instrument (such as the pointed end of a Mitchell's trimmer) to press on to the buccal plate, and it will perforate over any bony defect. If this proves impossible (and this is unusual) then clinical judgement together with radiographic interpretation should be used to estimate the position of the apex of the tooth. Bone removal begins at that point. Bone removal continues until good visibility and access are obtained. The minimum amount of bone consistent with these objectives is removed. Once the apical portion of the tooth is exposed the next phase begins.

Apicectomy

This part of the procedure may be performed using visual magnification if this is available. In order to maximise the support for the tooth at the end of surgery only the minimum amount of tooth consistent with the removal of the apical abnormality and associated pathology should be excised (Fig 7-6c). The angle of cut should be as close as possible to 90° to the long axis of the root to reduce the area of exposed dentine tubules. This can be achieved either by grinding down from the apex or by choosing a point in the root at which a fissure bur is inserted and advanced through the thickness of the root to remove the apical portion in one piece. The advantage of the latter method is that it allows inspection of the excised portion, which can inform the clinician of the completeness of removal. In other words, it is easy to inspect the full circumference of the root surface. In addition, inspection of the excised section will reveal the pattern of the canal at the apex. This provides useful information prior to retrograde root filling. The other method of grinding down the apex does not allow this, and it is possible to leave shavings of root deep in the surgical site, especially in the palatal/lingual aspect. This method is preferred, however, if working in the region of the maxillary sinus, as splitting off of an apex in such situations may result in the fragment entering the antrum.

Curettage

Any soft tissue lesion should be removed and ideally sent for histopathological examination. A number of pathological processes may present as periapical radiolucencies. These may include keratocysts (Fig 7-10), brown tumours of hyperparathyroidism and even malignancy. Curettage of the surgical site is continued until a clean bony surface is present.

Apical Seal

When the apicectomy has exposed a well-condensed root filling then no other seal is required. If an apical seal is required, it is necessary to complete a preparation for the filling material. This can be achieved by using a small round bur in a miniature handpiece or by use of sonic or ultrasonic instruments (Figs 7-6d and 7-8). Visual magnification is useful at this stage.

The material used to produce the apical seal has changed over the years. Amalgam is no longer considered acceptable, and a variety of materials are in current use.

Materials such as intermediate restorative material (IRM (Fig 7-6e) or mineral trioxide aggregate (MTA) are useful. When placing the seal, it is obvious that the field should be as dry as possible. The bony cavity can be obturated with a number of different materials. Bone wax is easy to handle but expensive, ribbon gauze is less costly. Once the seal has been placed the area is irrigated thoroughly, the material obturating the bony defect is removed and further irrigation is performed.

Wound Closure

Unless a vertical incision has been used the wound is closed with sutures (Fig 7-6f). Suture gauges of 3/0 or 4/0 are recommended. Some clinicians prefer to use monofilament non-resorbable sutures to reduce wicking of bacteria into the wound. When non-resorbable sutures are used they should be removed in three to four days. A variety of types of suturing can be used (see Chapter 3). Single interrupted sutures are useful in vertical incisions. Vertical mattress or modified sling sutures (Fig 7-9) are useful in pulling the gingival margin around the teeth, especially when the teeth are crowned. When a horizontal incision has been used a continuous suture can be employed.

When suturing is complete the wound should be compressed with damp gauze for three to five minutes. As mentioned elsewhere in this book, it is important that the patient is not discharged until haemostasis has been achieved.

Occlusion

It is important to assess the occlusion on the tooth to be operated on prior to surgery. The tooth should not be subjected to heavy loads post-opera-

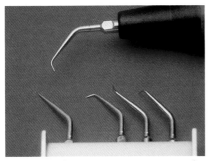

Fig 7-8 Ultrasonic instruments can be used to prepare a site for a retrograde root filling.

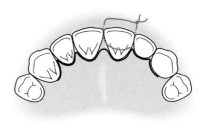

Fig 7-9 The modified sling suture.

tively, especially during the initial healing period. It may be necessary to adjust the occlusion both pre-operatively and in the event of passive eruption.

Post-operative Pain Control

Post-operative pain will occur after apical surgery unless analgesics are taken. As mentioned in Chapter 4, pre-emptive dosing is preferred. Most patients will experience some discomfort both on the day and the day after surgery. It is therefore worthwhile recommending that patients take analgesia until the day after surgery. A non-steroidal-inflammatory drug such as ibuprofen (400mg three times daily) is ideal. When non-steroidals are contraindicated paracetamol (up to 1g four times daily) is recommended.

Review

The patient should be reviewed at one week to assess healing. The area is inspected for swelling, discharge and tooth mobility. The patient should be questioned about any discomfort or bad taste. Sutures can be removed at this stage and the taking of a radiograph to establish a baseline view of bone loss is recommended at this visit. A further review may be made one to three months later. At this time complete healing of the soft tissues should have occurred. At this visit the area is inspected for the presence of a persistent sinus, swelling and tooth mobility. Further reviews including radiographic assessment are performed at six and 12 months. Large defects may require monitoring over extended periods. Further radiographs should be taken no more than annually until a stable or healed view is obtained. Occasionally a

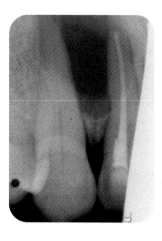

Fig 7-10 A keratocyst mimicking periapical infection at an upper lateral incisor.

persistent, symptomless radiolucency is apparent radiographically. As long as the defect does not increase in size it can be left alone, as it often comprises scar tissue connecting buccal and lingual bony defects.

Troubleshooting

Apical surgery may fail. The first factor to consider is: was apical surgery the correct treatment for this patient? In other words, the diagnosis of the problem must be correct. Conditions that may be confused with periapical infection include other bony lesions (Fig 7-10), periodontal conditions and fractured roots. In addition, pulpal or periapical pathology may be present in a neighbouring tooth Thus it is wise to pulp-test adjacent teeth before performing apical surgery. Another useful tip is to place a radio-opaque marker such as a gutta percha point into any sinus present before taking a radiograph (Fig 7-11). It is often difficult to diagnose a fractured root, especially when the defect runs mesiodistally (Fig 7-12) rather than buccolingually (Fig 7-13). Fractured roots must be considered, in particular in teeth with large posts supporting crowns.

Other reasons for failure include coronal leakage subsequent to surgery. This may occur some time after surgery if the coronal restoration begins to fail in clinical service.

If initially successful apical surgery fails on a tooth with an excellent root treatment and a sound coronal seal, then one wonders if the procedure should

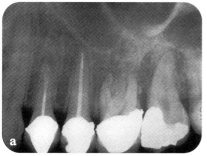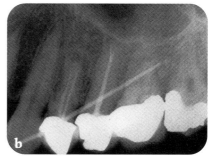

Fig 7-11 (a) Radiograph of a patient referred for apicectomy to upper premolar teeth. (b) A gutta percha point inserted into the buccal sinus revealed the source of the infection to be the upper first molar tooth.

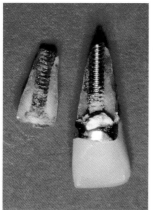

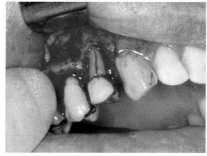

Fig 7-12 The fractured root of an upper central incisor. The fracture was discovered during an apicectomy.

Fig 7-13 The vertical root fracture in this upper premolar is obvious once the flap has been raised.

be repeated. Repeating surgery, using conventional approaches only, succeeds in about one-third of cases.

Lateral Perforation Repair

The technique of lateral repair is similar to that described for apicectomy (Fig 7-14). The only difference relates to bone removal. The bone is often replaced with a soft tissue lesion in the area of interest, and this exposes the perforation (Fig 7-14a). If sufficient access is not present it is achieved by

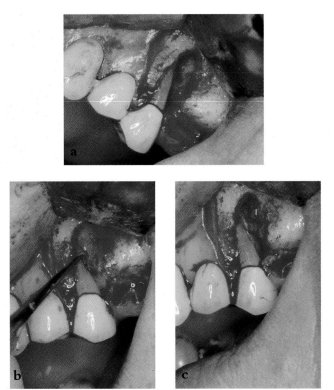

Fig 7-14 (a) A lateral perforation of the root of this upper premolar has caused extensive bone loss. (b) The perforation is modified with an ultrasonic tip. (c) The retrograde root filling in the perforation (in this case amalgam was used but this is no
longer recommended).

gradually removing bone around the area of the perforation. The apex of the
tooth is not exposed. As with apicectomy, bone removal should be conservative to provide good post-operative support and prevent damage to important structures.

Once the perforation has been exposed it can be modified with a bur or ultrasonic or sonic instrumentation before filling (Fig 7-14b). Alternatively, it
may be obturated without adjustment. The materials used for retrograde fill-
ings are employed.

Wound closure, post-operative care and follow-up are as described above
for apicectomy.

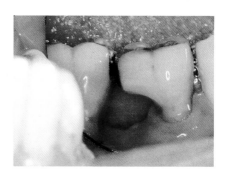

Fig 7-15 A lower molar that has had a root resected, the furcation is located coronally.

Root Resection

Occasionally, it is impossible to satisfactorily treat one root of a multi-rooted tooth by conventional endodontics or apicectomy. This may be due to extreme dilacerations or localised periodontal disease. In such cases, it is possible to remove the involved root while maintaining the remaining root(s). This is only recommended when the furcation is located coronally (Fig 7-15).

The procedure is as follows: first, the pulp chamber and roots that are to be maintained are obturated with endodontic filling material. Next the root to be removed is separated from the rest of the tooth using a fissure bur attached to a surgical handpiece. This separated root is then elevated from its socket with care to avoid damage to the remaining tooth. Elevation is often all that is required, as roots condemned for resection are often associated with periodontal disease. If the root does not elevate easily, a mucoperiosteal flap and careful bone removal with burs are needed (Fig 7-16).

Once the resected root is removed the defect in the remaining tooth is filled with a conventional restorative material and contoured to allow good oral hygiene. If oral hygiene is going to be difficult, then hemisection of the tooth is preferred, followed by provision of a crown.

Conclusions

- Apicectomy is not an alternative to sound conventional endodontics.
- Apicectomy is occasionally indicated.
- Lateral root perforation can be treated by endodontic surgery.

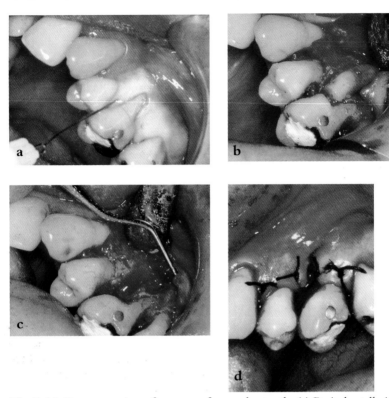

Fig 7-16 Root resection of an upper first molar tooth. (a) Periodontally involved mesiobuccal root is obvious. (b) Mesio-buccal root separated from tooth by use of a fissure bur in a handpiece. (c) Mesiobuccal root removed. (d) Wound closure.

Further Reading

Bell GW. A study of the suitability of referrals for periradicular surgery. Br Dent J 1998;184:183-6.

Chong BS. Managing Endodontic Failure in Practice. London: Quintessence, 2004.

Peterson J, Gutmann JL. The outcome of endodontic resurgery: a systematic review. Int Endodont J 2001;34:169-175.

Chapter 8
Surgery as an Aid to Orthodontics

Aim

This chapter will describe techniques that can be used to aid the eruption and movement of teeth.

Outcome

After reading this chapter you will have an understanding of the surgical techniques available to aid orthodontics.

Introduction

When planning minor oral surgery in combination with orthodontics, it is important to coordinate treatment with the clinician performing the tooth movement, which may vary. An example is the exposure of a palatally placed unerupted permanent maxillary canine (see below). Some orthodontists advocate maintenance of the deciduous canine, while others prefer the deciduous tooth to be removed at the time of the exposure.

Minor oral surgery can help orthodontics in many ways. The following are some examples:
- exposure of unerupted teeth
- attachment of orthodontic appliances to unerupted teeth
- removal of obstructions to orthodontic movement
- placement of anchorage
- tooth transplantation.

Exposure of Unerupted Teeth

There are two basic techniques of exposure. These are:
- tissue sacrifice (open exposure)
- flap reposition (closed exposure).

These methods may be employed alone or in combination with extraction - for example, of a preceding deciduous tooth. The choice between

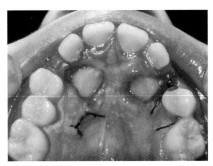

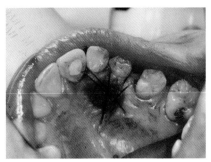

Fig 8-1 Two upper permanent canine teeth that were exposed by soft tissue sacrifice and bone removal. The suture on the patient's right side was used to arrest haemorrhage from the greater palatine artery. The sutures on the left were used to replace a small palatal flap that was raised to remove a palatally positioned ectopic second premolar, performed at the same time as the canine exposures.

Fig 8-2 Ribbon gauze soaked in Whitehead's varnish and held in position with sutures, used as a pack over an exposed maxillary canine.

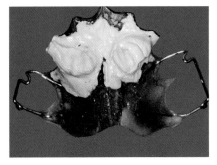

Fig 8-3 Coe-Pak on an upper removable appliance used as packs to cover the canines exposed in Fig 8-1.

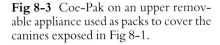

the two exposure methods depends upon the position of the unerupted tooth.

The position of the unerupted tooth is established by:
• clinical examination
• parallax radiography.

Clinical examination may detect bulges over unerupted crowns. In addition, the tipping of adjacent teeth can often offer clues to the position of an unerupted tooth. If the crown of an upper lateral incisor is tipped palatally, it suggests that an unerupted canine is palatal, as it is pushing the incisor root buccally.

A number of radiographic techniques can be used to localise buried teeth. The most useful examples are two periapical views taken at different angulations or panoramic and occlusal views. A panoramic view may provide information on its own by comparison of the two sides. Teeth closer to the X-ray tube (that is teeth placed palatally) appear larger on the film.

If the crown of the unerupted tooth is covered by attached gingiva, such as the palatal mucosa, then simple tissue sacrifice followed by bone removal is normally sufficient (Fig 8-1). Palatal tissue sacrifice can occasionally produce significant bleeding, as part of the incision may cut the greater palatine artery. This is easily controlled by passing a suture across the posterior part of the wound (Fig 8-1). The defect in the gingiva or palatal mucosa is best packed to prevent early tissue overgrowth. In addition, this may aid patient comfort. A variety of packs may be used, such as ribbon gauze soaked in White-head's varnish (Fig 8-2), a periodontal dressing such as Coe-Pak or bone wax. These may be held in place by sutures or, if a dressing material or bone wax is used, they can be added to a cover plate or removable orthodontic appliance (Fig 8-3). When held in place by sutures, the pack should be removed about seven to 10 days post-operatively. If the pack is added to an appliance it can be maintained indefinitely.

When the crown of the tooth is located under reflected mucosa or when tissue sacrifice would involve part of the wound margin including reflected

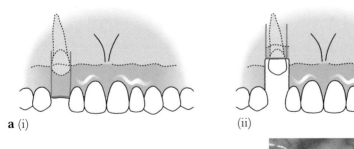

a (i)   (ii)

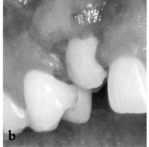

Fig 8-4 (a) An apically repositioned flap: i) Outline of flap ii) Flap repositioned apically to provide a collar of attached gingiva around the exposed tooth. (b) Clinical appearance of an apically repositioned flap used to expose a maxillary canine one week after surgery.

mucosa, another exposure technique should be chosen. This may involve the attachment of orthodontic appliances as described below. Alternatively, flap repositioning may be used. In this technique, once the flap has been raised it is repositioned apically to its original location (Fig 8-4). This produces a cuff of attached gingiva at the cervical margin of the exposed tooth. In the early post-operative phase the gingival margin can be quite bulky (Fig 8-4b), but this resolves with time. If this method compromises the gingival margins of neighbouring erupted teeth, it should not be used and one of the methods described later should be selected.

Attachment of Orthodontic Appliances to Unerupted Teeth

A number of different devices can be attached to unerupted teeth to allow orthodontic traction to be applied. These include:
* stainless steel wires and ligatures
* orthodontic brackets
* gold chains (Fig 8-5)
* magnets (Fig 8-6).

Since the introduction of etching techniques the last three methods are preferred. The method is as follows:
1) Any necessary extractions in the area of surgery are performed.
2) A mucoperiosteal flap is raised (Fig 8-5b). The incision includes the point of eruption of the tooth (or the socket edge of the above extraction sites if this is the point of eruption).
3) Bone is removed to expose the crown of the unerupted tooth (Fig 8-5c).
4) The crown is prepared for bonding, bearing in mind that high-pressure air-drying must be avoided. This is to prevent surgical emphysema. A dry 10 or 20ml syringe may be used to aid drying (Fig 8-5d).
5) The tooth is bonded in the normal manner (Fig 8-5e). The use of a moisture-insensitive primer is advised.
6) The bracket, chain or magnet is attached to the tooth by using a resin composite material (Fig 8-5f,g).
7) The flap is closed. When a chain has been attached, the free end of the chain may be bonded to an adjacent erupted tooth or sutured to mucosa (Fig 8-5h).

When using chains it is advised to pass a suture through the chain to prevent loss via the aspirator. When using magnets it is important to mark the poles (Fig 8-6c) so that, when aligned, they attract and do not repel. The magnet opposite that attached to the tooth is incorporated into a denture or removable appliance (Fig 8-6d).

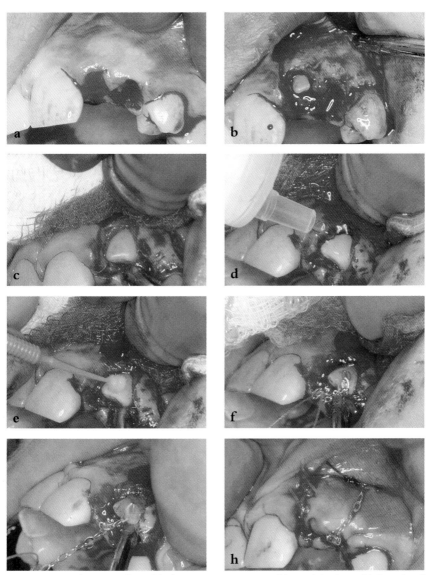

Fig 8-5 Attachment of a gold chain to an unerupted lateral incisor. (a) Retained upper left deciduous lateral incisor and canine teeth removed. (b) Flap raised. (c) Bone removed to expose permanent lateral incisor. (d) 20ml syringe used to dry tooth. (e) Etching of the exposed tooth. (f) Gold chain being positioned (note the chain is attached to a suture to prevent loss via suction or via pharynx). (g) Chain attached with composite resin. (h) Chain sutured to mucosa and wound closure.

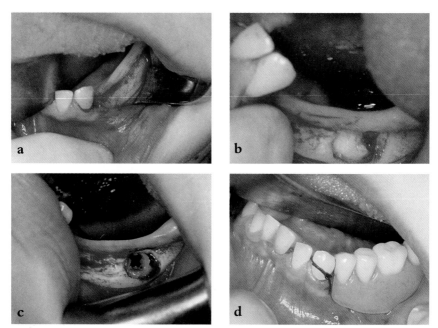

Fig 8-6 Attachment of a magnet to an ectopic lower premolar tooth. (a) Flap raised. (b) Bone removed to expose tooth. (c) Magnet attached to tooth with acid etch composite resin. Note the mark on the magnet denoting the side to be placed occlusally. (d) The opposite pole of the magnet is placed in a partial denture.

Removal of Obstructions to Orthodontic Movement

Obstructions to the movement of teeth may be either:

- hard tissue
- soft tissue.

Hard tissue may be:

- bone
- teeth
- other dental tissue
  - supernumerary teeth
  - odontomes.

The removal of bone alone is an unusual procedure. It will normally be undertaken in association with exposure or application of an orthodontic device as described above. The removal of teeth has been described in Chapters 5 and 6. One point worth remembering is that when removing unerupted teeth to allow the eruption of another unerupted tooth it is important to expose the crowns of both. This aids identification.

The removal of supernumerary teeth and odontomes follows the techniques described for tooth removal. The surgical options were discussed in Chapter 6. There are four treatment options for unerupted teeth as part of an orthodontic treatment plan.
These are:
• maintain and review
• surgical exposure
• transplantation
• surgical removal.

If the tooth is to be maintained it should be established that it is not going to interfere with orthodontic movement of neighbouring teeth. If exposure is considered then it must be determined that orthodontic alignment is possible.

The removal of soft tissue to allow eruption has been described above in relation to unerupted teeth. One area of soft tissue that might interfere with tooth movement is a fraenum, especially in the maxillary mid-line. Such fraenae do not always produce problems, although they are often associated with a diastema. It is best to await the eruption of permanent maxillary canines before performing a fraenectomy, as the space may close spontaneously. Before performing a fraenectomy as an aid to diastema closure it is important to exclude other causes of diastema, such as a mesiodens, by taking appropriate radiographs. The techniques of fraenectomy for a maxillary midline fraenum and a lingual fraenum, which may cause ankyloglossia (tongue-tie), are described below.

Maxillary midline fraenectomy
This procedure is illustrated in Fig 8-7. It can be performed with a scalpel, diathermy or laser. When using a scalpel an elliptical incision is made along the length of the fraenum (Fig 8-7a). A minimal amount of mucosa is removed, but all underlying muscle attachment is excised. A stay suture is inserted at the sulcus reflection to anchor the mucosa to periosteum (Fig 8-7b). This maintains sulcus depth. If the fraenum is inserted into the palatal mucosa the small zone of attached gingiva on the palatal side is sacrificed. The labial wound is closed with sutures, and a pack such as Coe-Pak can be placed in the interdental and palatal defect.

Lingual fraenectomy
This procedure is used to correct tongue-tie and is illustrated in Fig 8-8. It

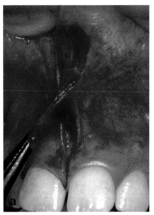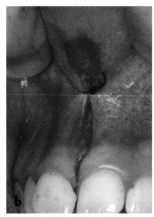

Fig 8-7 Maxillary midline fraenectomy. (a) Elliptical incision with removal of minimal mucosa but all of underlying muscle attachment. (b) Insertion of stay suture at sulcus reflection to anchor mucosa to periosteum and maintain sulcus depth.

differs from that described above for maxillary fraenectomy. This time the incision is made in a horizontal direction (Fig 8-8b). Normally no tissue is removed (Fig 8-8c). However, some clinicians excise a triangular section of the fraenum. It is important to note the position of the submandibular ducts so that these are not damaged by the incision or when suturing the wound at the end of the procedure (Fig 8-8d).

Placement of Anchorage

Occasionally there is not sufficient tooth anchorage available to allow the application of the appropriate forces to allow the orthodontic movement. This is often the case in patients with hypodontia. Additional anchorage can be obtained with extra-oral traction. Alternatively intra-oral techniques can be used. These employ the use of implants or bone plates to supply the anchorage. These implants may be standard dental implants or those designed specifically for orthodontic movement.

Implants designed for anchorage are normally placed in the midline of the palate (Fig 8-9). They are much smaller than dental implants and are used to anchor orthodontic appliances such as transpalatal bars. The implants are removed after orthodontic treatment.

Tooth Transplantation

Tooth transplantation is a useful means of aiding orthodontic treatment, as

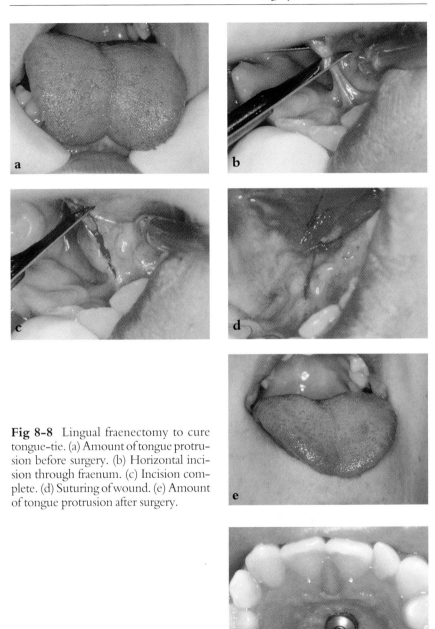

Fig 8-8 Lingual fraenectomy to cure tongue-tie. (a) Amount of tongue protrusion before surgery. (b) Horizontal incision through fraenum. (c) Incision complete. (d) Suturing of wound. (e) Amount of tongue protrusion after surgery.

Fig 8-9 A palatal implant used as orthodontic anchorage.

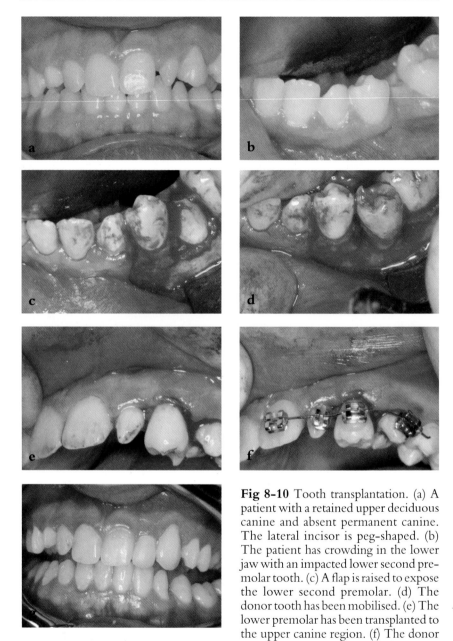

Fig 8-10 Tooth transplantation. (a) A patient with a retained upper deciduous canine and absent permanent canine. The lateral incisor is peg-shaped. (b) The patient has crowding in the lower jaw with an impacted lower second premolar tooth. (c) A flap is raised to expose the lower second premolar. (d) The donor tooth has been mobilised. (e) The lower premolar has been transplanted to the upper canine region. (f) The donor tooth has been splinted to the adjacent teeth with orthodontic brackets and wire. (g) The appearance after crowning of the peg shaped lateral incisor and donor tooth.

it can achieve something beyond the skills of even the best orthodontic practitioner - namely it is a method of moving teeth between the jaws. Transplantation can be used to achieve two goals:
• transplantation of an ectopic tooth to its natural position
• transplantation of a tooth to another site (Fig 8-10).

The surgical technique for both is similar. Before describing the surgical technique it is worth considering two points. First, the ideal time to transplant a tooth is when its root formation is two-thirds to three-quarters complete. Secondly, it is possible to move transplanted teeth orthodontically.

The surgical technique is as follows:
1) Administer prophylactic antibiotics such as a single 3g dose of amoxicillin orally at the start of the procedure.
2) Remove the donor tooth. This must be performed as atraumatically as possible. It is especially important to avoid unnecessary damage to the periodontal ligament. If the donor tooth is erupted then a number 11 blade should be run around the gingival margin to cut the marginal periodontal fibres (Fig 8-11). In order to avoid further contact with the root of the tooth the tooth should be removed by the crown. This is the opposite of the standard approach to dental extractions. A way of achieving this is to place a dental cotton wool roll over the tooth before application of the forceps (Fig 8-12). In addition this protects the crown against damage from the beaks of the forceps.
3) Once the tooth has been mobilised it should be replaced in its original socket until it is time for transplantation.
4) Preparation of the recipient site can begin once the donor has been mobilised. This should not be performed until it is apparent that the donor is suitable. If a tooth is present at the recipient site it is extracted. If the

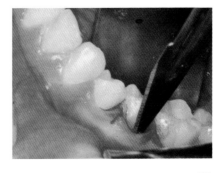

Fig 8-11 When an erupted tooth is used as a donor a scalpel blade is run around the marginal periodontium to aid atraumatic extraction.

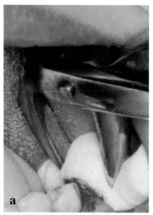
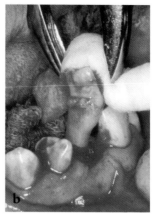

Fig 8-12 When removing a donor tooth for transplantation the tooth should be protected from damage by protecting it with a cotton wool roll.

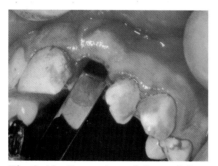
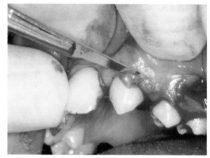

Fig 8-13 Expansion of the recipient socket with a chisel.

Fig 8-14 Modification of the gingival margin around a transplanted maxillary canine.

socket is not the correct shape, it needs to be modified. Deepening and expanding the socket with a chisel without raising a mucoperiosteal flap can achieve this (Fig 8-13). If there is no socket at the donor site then a mucoperiosteal flap is raised. Inserting chisels vertically at the mesial and distal aspects of the recipient site makes a bony flap. These are then joined with a bone cut along the ridge. The resultant bone flap is elevated in a buccal direction. The depth of the socket can be adjusted using a chisel. Occasionally, it is possible to have a choice of teeth to transplant. An example is when two lower premolars are being removed and one is being used to replace an upper central incisor. In such cases one of the potential donors (the less favourable of the two) is used as a template to assess the 'fit' of the donor in the socket. This minimises the trauma to the periodontal ligament of the prime donor tooth.

5) The donor tooth is placed in the recipient site.

6) If necessary, the gingiva is recontoured with a scalpel blade (Fig 8-14).

7) Sutures are placed around the donor to ensure good gingival apposition.

8) If necessary, the donor tooth is stabilised by bonding to an orthodontic wire attached to neighbouring teeth or as part of a fixed orthodontic appliance.

9) The donor tooth should undergo pulp extirpation after two weeks, at which time calcium hydroxide is placed in the canal.

10) The temporary root-filling material is replaced at three-monthly intervals, and if progress is satisfactory the definitive root treatment is performed at one year.

As mentioned above, the transplanted tooth can be moved orthodontically, if this is required. This can begin three months after transplantation. It may be necessary if there is insufficient bone at the ideal site for the transplant. If this is the case the transplanted tooth is placed as close as possible to the ideal position and then moved orthodontically.

Alteration of the crown of the transplanted tooth is necessary if it is has been moved into a site other than its natural position in the arch - for example, a lower premolar into an upper central incisor socket.

Conclusions

Minor oral Surgery can aid orthodontics by exposing teeth, removing obstructions to tooth movement and by tooth transplantation.

Further Reading

Andreasen JO, Paulsen HU, Yu Z, Schwartz O. A long-term study of 370 autotransplanted premolars. Part II. Tooth survival and pulp healing subsequent to transplantation. Eur J Orthod 1990;12:14-24.

Andreasen JO, Paulsen HU, Yu Z, Schwartz O. A long-term study of 370 autotransplanted premolars. Part III. Periodontal healing subsequent to transplantation. Eur J Orthod 1990;12:25-37.

Blair GS, Hobson RS, Leggat TG. Post-treatment assessment of surgically exposed and orthodontically aligned impacted maxillary canines. Am J Orthod Dentofacial Orthop 1998;113:329-332.

Chapter 9

Implants and Surgery to Facilitate Prosthetic Dentistry

Aim

This chapter describes some basic surgical techniques that can be applied to facilitate the functional and aesthetic replacement of missing teeth and the selection of patients for implant treatment.

Outcome

After reading this chapter you should:
- have a basic understanding of how surgery can aid, or sometimes hinder, the successful rehabilitation of patients who have lost or are about to lose teeth.
- be aware of surgical techniques that can be used to improve the function and aesthetics of fixed and removable prostheses.
- appreciate the role that hard and soft tissues play in achieving restoration of the dentition with good aesthetics.
- be able to assess patients for implant treatment from a surgical aspect.

Introduction

The majority of our patients expect to keep their natural teeth for life. Trauma, dental disease and congenital abnormalities can result in the loss of teeth and the need for their replacement. The support of an adequate residual alveolar ridge is helpful for the stability, retention and appearance of fixed and removable prostheses. Following tooth loss, alveolar resorption begins and continues throughout life. Many patients with removable prostheses can adapt to this situation. Others will benefit from a variety of surgical techniques to 'turn back time' and restore the supporting tissues. Dental implant systems and techniques developed in the latter half of the 20th century enable dentists to replace missing teeth and predictably improve masticatory function. The scope and need for conventional 'preprosthetic' surgery has changed with this revolution in dental care. This chapter will define techniques that still have a place in the 21st century to modify the hard and soft tissues of the mouth in order to improve the provision and patient acceptance of dental prostheses and facilitate the use of dental implants.

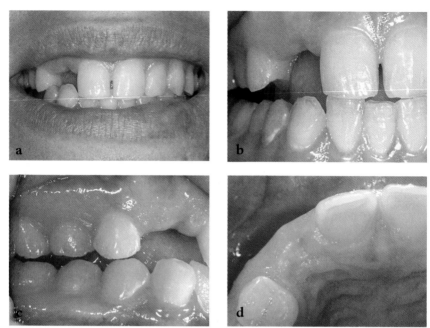

Fig 9-1 Planning photographs for implant replacement of the upper right lateral incisor. (a) Front view with smile note aesthetics and symmetry of soft issues. (b) Teeth in protrusion. (c) Right lateral guidance. (d) Occlusal view to assess ridge width.

Rehabilitation of Patients who are Undergoing Exodontia

Surgical planning undertaken prior to the removal of a tooth or teeth should take into account the consequences for prosthetic replacement and how this might be accomplished. It is unusual to plan the removal of a functional tooth in isolation; the majority of patients will require careful consideration of how their dentition can be preserved and rehabilitated in the light of their future functional and aesthetic needs.

Details of tooth form, aesthetics, soft-tissue contour, appearance, symmetry and smile line together with jaw relationship (if appropriate) should be recorded using clinical photographs, shade guides and study casts (Fig 9-1a-d). This information, together with a diagnostic wax up of the proposed restoration, can prove invaluable to both the dentist and technician in planning care and explaining the proposed treatment to the patient. It is also important to ask the simple question as to why exodontia is required. This will inform preventative measures. It may lead to strategies to avoid further tooth loss and aid preservation of existing hard and soft-tissue topography.

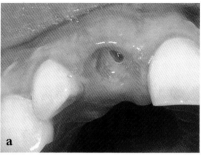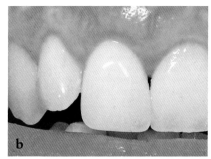

Fig 9-2 (a) Preservation of soft tissue topography after fitting a correctly adjusted socket fitted partial denture prior to implant placement. (b) Denture in place.

Strategies to Facilitate Prosthetic Rehabilitation at the Time of Exodontia

The following should be considered at the time of extraction:
- analysis of the reasons for exodontia
- prevention of further unplanned tooth loss
- preservation of existing dental information by making good historical records
- preservation of soft tissue topography by temporary support by:
  - retaining tooth roots in the absence of pathology
  - using socket fitted dentures (Fig 9-2) or placement of correctly contoured bridge pontics
  - placing immediate implants to support gingival papillae
- preservation of existing hard tissues by:
  - retaining healthy tooth roots to preserve bone volume and ridge shape – roots can be used as over-denture supports or submerged to act as ridge maintainers
  - immediate placement of dental implants
  - atraumatic extraction techniques (use of periotomes to cut the periodontal ligament and deliver the tooth root)
  - care in post-operative digital socket compression so as not to unduly reduce alveolar width
  - osteoplastic flaps to maintain the alveolar bone (a composite flap of cortical plate with attached soft tissues giving 'trap door' access to the buried tooth that can be repositioned to restore ridge contour)
  - grafting of the extraction socket to preserve alveolar bone.

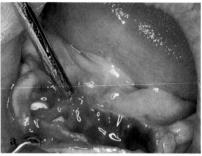
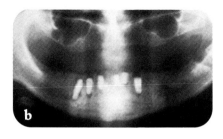

Fig 9-3 (a) Placement of ceramic cones to preserve clinical ridge topography. (b) Immediate radiograph.

- hydroxyapatite cones or granules can be effective at physically maintaining local alveolar bone width and height improving support for a lower denture (Fig 9-3).
- if implants are contemplated at a future date, sockets can be filled with material to act as an osteoconductive scaffold to facilitate new bone formation; examples include artificial materials such as calcium carbonate or tricalcium phosphate granules, which are resorbed and replaced by new bone. Osteoinductive agents that act both as a scaffold and to stimulate bone cells locally can also be used, examples being demineralised human bone matrix, freeze-dried deproteinised bovine bone, autologous bone harvested from the patient and genetically engineered bone morphogenic proteins.
• Circumspection in the application of techniques to contour the alveolus.

When teeth are lost, resorption of the associated alveolar bone begins and continues inexorably, although at a decreased rate after the first year. There is thus little justification for the unnecessary removal of bone at the time of exodontia. The resorption process also makes predicting the outcome of any surgical intervention difficult. The reduction of bony undercuts should be limited to those essential to facilitate denture insertion. The use of an anterior buccal flange on a denture to aid retention can be difficult where a prominent buccal undercut exists. In such circumstances the situation is usually best dealt with by providing an open-faced or socketed denture and reassessing the situation after a few months. This approach also aids preservation of soft-tissue topography.

Surgical Techniques Facilitating Prosthodontic Rehabilitation

Surgery can be used to correct unfavourable hard and soft-tissue relationships to enable a more stable and retentive prosthesis to be produced. Some of this surgery, such as osteotomies to correct gross skeletal discrepancies in facial form, falls outwith the scope of minor oral surgery. Other operations - for example, simple soft-tissue procedures to reduce muscle attachments and improve the peripheral seal of prostheses - are amenable to outpatient practice. The aim of surgery is to enable the provision of a prosthesis that will:

- restore function (mastication, speech and deglutition)
- be stable
- be retentive
- preserve the remaining dental structures
- satisfy the patient's aesthetic requirements
- give the patient 'dental confidence'.

Surgery has been advocated to build up the alveolar bone and deepen the buccal and lingual sulci to mitigate the effects of alveolar resorption. This restores clinical ridge height, so improving the foundation for denture construction. The techniques used in this type of surgery have, in the main, fallen into disuse due to their high morbidity, requirement for hospital support and the effects of inexorable alveolar resorption negating any temporary improvement in ridge height that could be achieved.

Techniques still in frequent use are covered below.

Specific Factors that Influence Care and Affect Planning for Surgery or Implants

The initial clinical presentation of a patient will determine whether their expectations are realistic and what prosthodontic outcome can be achieved from the baseline position.

The medical status of the patient exerts a major influence. Conditions that affect the patient's capacity to withstand surgical intervention and healing are important. Any specific local or systemic problems that influence the response of the hard and soft tissues to surgery will affect the prognosis. Such factors include sclerotic or osteoporotic bone, local infection and any pre-existing pathology.

The occlusion, skeletal relationships and local anatomy (inferior alveolar nerve, maxillary sinus, floor of nose, tongue size) will influence planning. Other factors that affect the management include parafunctional habits, oral hygiene and the use of tobacco. An obvious factor that is important is the degree of coop-

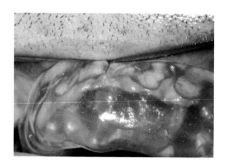

Fig 9-4 Use of a guide or stent, made on a copy of the master model to replicate the fitting surface of the denture, placed following recontouring of the ridge – blood acts as 'pressure relieving paste' to indicate bony prominences requiring relief of denture or further smoothing.

eration that can be achieved. It is useful, during planning and to inform the consent process, to consider that patients are somewhere on a slope - those who are fully fit with good oral hygiene, adequate alveolar bone and ideal soft tissues being at the top of the slope, with the best prognosis for a successful functional and aesthetic outcome. Factors elucidated during the history taking and examination will determine where a particular patient is on the 'success slope', and by weighing local and systemic factors the clinician and patient will gain an appreciation of the likely clinical outcome. It also enables the clinician to demonstrate to the patient how modification of factors (e.g. giving up smoking, improving oral hygiene, grafting alveolar bone, accepting a removable rather than a fixed restoration) can move them up the slope and improve prognosis.

Procedures to Improve the Peripheral Seal of Complete Prostheses

The following procedures can be used to aid denture retention:

Removal of Undercuts

Contouring of the jaw involves exposure of the bone, taking care to position the mucoperiosteal flaps. Margins should be supported by sound bone to reduce any shrinkage and loss of sulcus depth. Bony excess or irregularity can then be smoothed using a well-cooled bur or a bone file. This procedure is useful to reduce exostoses, tori and smooth irregular ridges or reduce prominent muscle attachments - for example, the mylohyoid ridge. Recontouring of the alveolus is facilitated by planning the desired reduction on a study model and producing a surgical guide – ideally to the predetermined fitting surface of the final prosthesis (Fig 9-4). At the time of surgery, the practitioner should always bear in mind that raising periosteum will stimulate bone resorption and that the main difficulty in placing implants is often lack of alveolar bone. Major recontouring of the alveolus and procedures such as alveolectomy and alveoplasty have fallen into disuse.

Smoothing of Sharp/ Knife-Edge Ridges

The oral mucosa can become traumatised between the fitting surface of a denture and an underlying knife-edge or serrated alveolar ridge. The provision of a resilient lining to the denture can ameliorate painful symptoms. Occasionally, however, limited smoothing of the ridge is beneficial.

Surgery to Prevent Trauma to Exposed Inferior Alveolar Nerves

As the alveolar bone is lost, the inferior alveolar nerve may come close to the crest of the ridge. The superficial position of the mental foramen can result in the mental nerve being traumatised by a lower denture. This may lead to intermittent pain. Surgical repositioning of the inferior alveolar nerve is possible but rarely indicated. The treatment of choice is to relieve the prosthesis in the area of the mental foramen and consider providing a tooth or implant supported rather than a tissue-borne prosthesis.

Removal of Fraenal Muscle Attachments

Attachment of muscles high on the ridge can result in displacement of dentures during speech and mastication. Denture flanges may traumatise such fraenae. Relieving the flanges to accommodate fraenae can also compromise the peripheral seal of the denture. The prosthesis is weakened at points of relief, and this may cause fracture of the denture.

Fraenal attachments can be removed using conventional surgery, electrosurgery or with the carbon dioxide laser. The aim is to restore the sulcus depth and leave attached mucosa in the denture-bearing area. The techniques are described in Chapter 8.

Removal of Excessive Soft Tissue/Flabby Ridges

The commonest area requiring soft-tissue reduction is the maxillary tuberosity. The technique can be applied to any area of unsupported soft tissue. It is important to consider the alternative of augmentation to recreate hard-tissue support. Surgery is based on removal of a double ellipse of tissue. The first incision is to remove excess tissue and a second undermining ellipse allows closure (Fig 9-5a-c).

Surgery to Increase the Size of the Denture Bearing Area

A number of procedures are used to increase the area available to support a denture. These are described as follows:

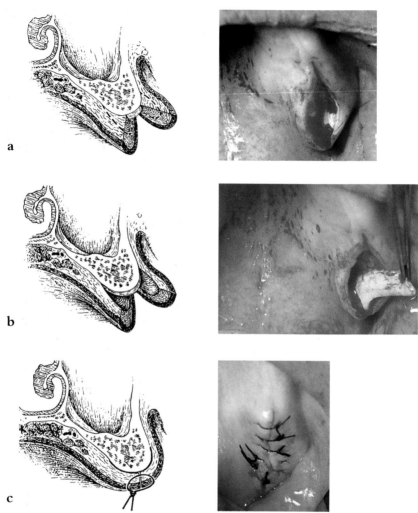

Fig 9-5 Double ellipse technique to reduce excess soft tissue and achieve primary closure. (a) Initial ellipse to remove excess. (b) Undermining ellipses to allow tension free closure. (c) Closure.

Sulcus-Deepening Procedures and Removal of Denture-Induced Hyperplasia

The buccal or lingual sulci can be deepened and reshaped using various recontouring 'vestibuloplasty' techniques. This enables extended denture flanges to be provided to improve retention and stability. The aim is to extend the clinical alveolar ridge height and eliminate the displacing effects of mus-

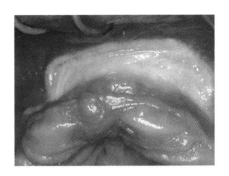

Fig 9-6 Appearance of sulcus in the upper anterior sextant following vestibuloplasty and repair using a split thickness skin graft.

cle attachments. To increase the size of the denture bearing area by modification of the soft tissues there needs to be sufficient residual alveolar bone. If deficient, augmentation of the alveolus may be required.

Many different vestibuloplasty techniques have been described. All aim to deepen the sulcus and provide attached mucosa onto which the prosthesis can be placed. The techniques rely on displacing muscle attachments apically to extend the denture-bearing area. The resultant denuded alveolus is left to granulate, or other techniques are used to reduce wound contraction and produce a stable tissue base for denture support. Inlay techniques in which the ridge was grafted using a free, split-thickness mucosal or skin graft were popular. Problems relating to lack of adequately sized donor sites, poor resilience of skin in the mouth and donor site morbidity have reduced the popularity of this approach (Fig 9-6).

Alternatives to grafting are laser vestibuloplasty, submucous vestibuloplasty, transposition of periosteum and mucosa, surgery to lower the floor of the mouth and use of pedicled muscle (temporalis) or mucosal/skin flaps. The latter techniques are reserved for post-cancer reconstruction and are outwith the sphere of minor oral surgery.

The development of soft-tissue surgery using the carbon dioxide laser has revolutionised intra-oral surgery in that large amounts of tissue can be removed with low morbidity and limited post-operative wound contraction. Vestibuloplasty and removal of extensive denture induced fibrous hyperplasia (caused by chronic trauma from ill-fitting denture flanges, following long-term denture wear and alveolar resorption) can be undertaken under local anaesthesia without grafting and with maintenance of sulcus depth.

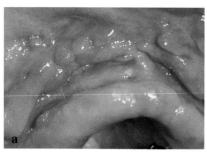 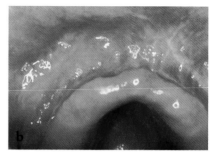

Fig 9-7 (a) Denture induced hyperplasia. (b) Sulcus following laser excision and vestibuloplasty.

In cases of denture-induced hyperplasia, dentures should be relieved. This will result in a reduction in trauma and inflammation. Small areas can then be excised conventionally or by electrosurgery. If the base is on attached mucosa, the wound can be left to granulate. If on mobile mucosa, the wound can be undermined and closed. In either case the sulcus is maintained. Extensive areas of hyperplastic tissue should be excised and the sulcus depth maintained by grafting or laser excision (Fig 9-7). Practitioners should always be wary of exophitic/hyperplastic lesions and consider the possibility of malignancy; all excised tissue should be sent for histopathological examination.

Alveolar Augmentation
Traumatic extractions, infection, periodontal disease and inappropriate loading of the bone by ill-fitting dentures or transmission of high occlusal loads from an opposing dentate arch can accelerate the process of bone loss.

Complex techniques and osteotomies (visor/sandwich) were used in the past to build up the jaw. Results were disappointing, however, in that little usable increase in clinical ridge height was achieved, even when a vestibuloplasty was undertaken. The act of surgery also renewed the vigour of the resorption process, leaving many patients no better off a few years after surgery. Augmentation of the alveolus, except for limited recontouring to fill in undercuts and reshape the ridge in pontic areas to improve hygiene and aesthetics, is almost exclusively related to preparing the jaws for implant placement.

Pre-implant Surgery
The hard and soft tissues have a major influence on the clinical outcome that can be achieved using implant-supported restorations. Adequate bone vol-

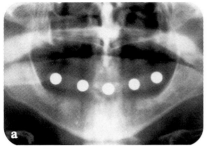 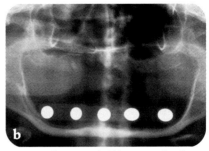

Fig 9-8 Two DPT radiographs, a stent with 7mm diameter ball bearings has been held in the mouth during exposure. (a) Adequate bone in the anterior mandible into which implants could be placed. (b) Less than 7mm of remaining mandibular bone.

ume (height and width) is required to enable implant placement in the correct position to support aesthetic and biomechanically sound restorations. Successful soft-tissue aesthetics depend on many factors, including the thickness, colour and quality of the attached gingivae, the tooth/implant position, angulation and presence of supporting bone.

Planning must also take account of anatomical structures such as the inferior alveolar neurovascular bundle, maxillary sinus, floor of nose and adjacent teeth. Planning of surgery thus requires analysis of appropriate radiographs to complement the physical examination. In the majority of cases standard radiographic techniques will confirm whether implant surgery is possible or not (Fig 9-8). It is in cases where there is doubt, or where surgery could affect vital structures, that more complex radiological investigations are required, such as computed tomography (CT) or other tomographic techniques (Fig 9-9). Three-dimensional CT reconstruction imaging can also assist surgery by enabling the production of surgical stents to guide the placement of implants of specific dimensions in predetermined positions, facilitating flapless surgery and immediate placement of prostheses (Fig 9-10).

Following examination, the need for any pre-implant surgery to enable implants to be placed in the correct position to achieve a good functional and aesthetic prosthesis will be determined. Not all patients will want, or be suitable for, more invasive surgical techniques. It should not be forgotten that excellent aesthetic results can be achieved by the use of techniques that employ artificial materials to replace lost tissues ('pink plastic') in association with implant-supported removable restorations.

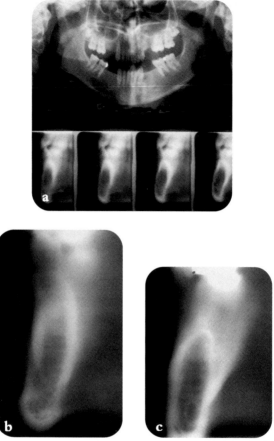

Fig 9-9 (a) Scanora dental tomograms taken for evaluation of the height and width of bone available above the mental foramen and inferior alveolar nerve when planning implants to replace congenitally missing lower premolars. (b) Detail showing mental nerve exiting from foramen. (c) Inferior alveolar canal.

Guided Bone Regeneration

In cases in which there are minimal defects of alveolar bone, allowing implant placement but lacking full coverage in bone, guided bone regeneration (GBR) techniques are helpful. GBR uses membranes as physical barriers to restrict the infiltration of soft tissues and encourage the formation of new bone in osseous defects. A variety of membranes are available for GBR. A non-resorbable material is expanded polytetrafluoroethylene.

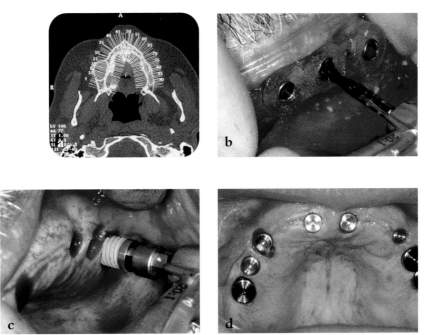

Fig 9-10 (a) Planning CT. (b) Stent in place guiding preparation of implant sites. (c) Implant being placed. (d) Implants in place.

Resorbable membranes are derived from synthetic and animal sources. The disadvantage of non-resorbable membranes is that they must be removed once bone formation is complete. In addition they are susceptible to becoming a nidus for infection. A benefit is that they protect the osseous defect for longer. Thus bone formation is more predictable compared to the use of resorbable membranes. GBR can be used alone or in combination with bone chips or bone substitutes to generate new bone around implants (Fig 9-11). GBR membranes are also used in association with onlay and other bone augmentation techniques to protect the graft site. They facilitate the revitalisation of harvested bone with reduced resorption.

Alveolar Bone Augmentation

There are a number of ways of increasing the hard tissue support for prostheses. These are described below:

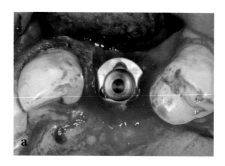

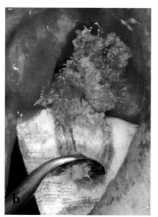
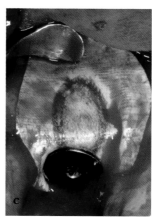

Fig 9-11 (a) Implant in place showing defect in buccal bone. (b) Expanded polytetrafluoroethylene membrane held aside to allow bone chips to be placed over exposed implant threads. (c) Membrane in place over defect.

Onlay Grafting

In the resorbed or damaged ridge, an onlay graft may be required to enable implant placement and optimise the final aesthetics. Fresh autogenous bone grafts have optimal osteoinductive properties in comparison with allogeneic, alloplastic or xenogenic grafts. The main disadvantage of autogenous bone grafts is associated with morbidity of the donor site. The amount of bone required at the prospective implant site often dictates the donor site. To augment a sextant of the alveolus, the mandibular symphysis or ramus are accessible and provide adequate volume (Fig 9-12). Extraoral donor site surgery for major grafts is unsuitable in general practice. Patients requiring such surgery should be referred to a maxillofacial surgeon. Onlay grafts can be used to increase ridge width and height, but it is important that once the graft has taken and the bone revitalised it is stimulated to prevent resorption. This is achieved

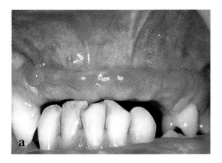
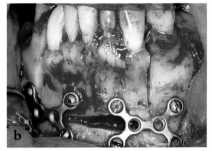

Fig 9-12 (a) Anterior maxilla – buccal concavity, limited inter-arch space. (b) Osteotomy to reposition lower anterior teeth to increase inter-arch space and harvest bone. (c) Onlay graft harvested from the mandibular symphysis, secured by temporary screws – implants can be placed in 4–5 months.

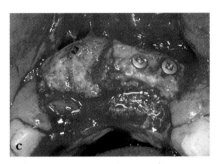

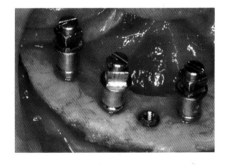

Fig 9-13 Onlay graft harvested from the anterior iliac crest secured to the atrophic mandible by immediate implants, prior to final contouring and soft tissue closure.

by placing implants three to six months after graft placement. Onlay grafts are usually performed using blocks of bone shaped and fixed to the residual alveolus, using screws or implants (Figs. 9-12 and 9-13). Bone chips and bone substitutes can be used if they can be protected from occlusal forces and supported by membranes and/or titanium mesh.

Ridge Expansion
The width of the residual alveolus can be widened by 'green stick'-fracturing apart the cortical plates. A midcrestal incision is made in a similar way to

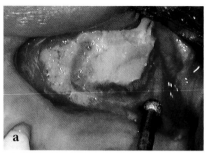
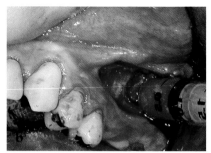

Fig 9-14 (a) Cutting of a trapdoor bone flap in the wall of the left sinus with a slow speed diamond bur. (b) Placement of compressed milled cortical bone trephined from the chin following infracture of trap door.

the 'osteoplastic flap technique'. The soft tissues are left attached and the cortical plates are fractured apart using chisels and osteotomes. This enables interpositional grafting material or immediate implants to be placed.

Sinus Augmentation
Bone quality and quantity are important variables affecting the success of implants. The posterior maxilla is known to have poor quality bone and often reduced volume because of pneumatisation by the maxillary sinuses. Onlay techniques can be used to increase ridge width or height, but if used for the latter there may be reduced interarch space for prosthetic restoration. Therefore, sinus augmentation procedures have been developed to overcome such problems.

Open Techniques
A modified Caldwell-Luc approach (Chapter 10) is utilised. A trapdoor is outlined in the lateral wall of the sinus using a water-cooled diamond bur, in order not to tear the sinus lining (Fig 9-14a). The trap door is then infractured, taking care to avoid perforation of the sinus-lining membrane (Fig 9-14b). This then forms the new, elevated floor of the sinus. Graft material is packed into the space. Particulate autogenous corticocancellous bone grafts are commonly used as the graft material. Adding artificial bone substitutes can expand the bone.

Closed Techniques
For local sinus augmentation it is possible to prepare an implant site, taking care not to penetrate the sinus floor, by up-fracturing the base of the site with socket-shaped osteotomes. The floor of the sinus can be gently raised

similar to pushing up a 'manhole' cover, bone chips are then pushed up through the implant site to create a 'mole hill' in the sinus floor into which the apex of the implant can be seated.

Distraction Techniques

Developed in the orthopaedic specialty, distraction techniques (where the bone is sectioned and the two parts slowly moved apart to stimulate new bone formation in the 'distraction gap') are now being applied to craniofacial and orthognathic surgery. The use of small intra-oral distraction devices can increase the bone volume, but usually in only one dimension at a time. This can be an alternative to guided bone regeneration or onlay grafting; these latter techniques often have to be used in conjunction with distraction to finally restore the contour of the alveolar ridge. Once in place the devices are activated daily (0.5–1mm) until the desired augmentation is achieved.

Implant Surgery

Modern surgical techniques for implant placement owe much to the pioneering work undertaken in the 1960s by innovators such as Per-Ingvar Brånemark, Andre Schroeder, Richard Skalak and George Zarb. Successful treatment, then as now, was dependent on the biological and biomechanical factors pertaining to the particular implant system used and on the surgical protocol employed in placing the implants. Implant systems and techniques have evolved since those early days. Nevertheless, practitioners should remember that every departure from the original protocols, with their long periods of undisturbed healing and delayed loading, requires even more rigour in the planning and selection of patients.

The stages of implant surgery vary depending upon the system used, but the following principles are common to the majority of systems:
- atraumatic surgery carried out under aseptic conditions:
  - appropriate use of antiseptic mouth rinses, gentle handling of soft tissues and appropriate flap design (margins on sound bone)
  - use of correct insertion torques, in particular, for tapered implants, to limit compression of the bone
- restrict the build up of frictional heat, keeping below the threshold of 47° C for one minute, above which osseointegration will be compromised
  - control of drill speed and torque and use of an intermittent drilling technique
  - use of irrigation to cool the drills and remove debris
  - use of sharp drills matched to the implants to be placed

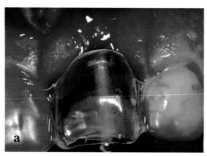 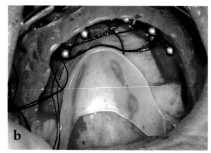

Fig 9-15 Surgical stents (with direction indicators in proposed implant sites) used to guide implant placement produced from diagnostic planning models or existing dentition. (a) For a single tooth. (b) For a full upper fixed bridge.

- preparation of wider diameter sites than normal in hard bone, and tapping of threads to reduce insertion torque
- placing implants to achieve high initial stability and thus enable early or immediate loading
  - in soft bone, stability can be enhanced by preparation of sites narrower than normal and not tapping threads
  - utilisation of mono- or bi-cortical fixation for short implants or in soft bone
- ensuring good soft-tissue aesthetics and health
  - placing implants with a minimum of 2mm of bone between implants and 3mm between an implant and a tooth will provide support for soft tissues and gingival papillae
  - appropriate use of implant supported crowns and pontics to restore missing teeth
  - selection of implant diameters to match crown widths to give good emergence profiles.
- placing sufficient implants in the correct positions to facilitate the restorative plan for rehabilitation
  - use of surgical stents to guide implant placement and determine position in the arch and in relation to the amelocemental junction of future crowns (Fig 9-15)
- maintaining primary stability
  - placement of implants ensuring the implant surface is not contaminated and its first contact is with the patients blood/bone
  - controlling forces applied to the implants during the healing period
  - correct implant placement to reduce the need for cantilevers and optimise force distribution

- implant placed to enable axial loading
- linking of implants to reduce micromovement.

Once integrated, implants are difficult to remove. Thus, care should be taken to ensure that the treatment provided is future-proof. The patient's circumstances will change over the years. Can the implant placed now for a single tooth be used to support a bridge or an overdenture? Can the transmucosal element be removed and the implant be put out of use? These issues, together with the type of restoration planned, the position in the arch, the quality of the tissues and the expertise of the implant team will determine the type of implant to be used.

Soft-Tissue Surgery

The techniques described below are used to modify the soft tissues prior to the provision of prostheses.

Free Grafts

Perioplastic procedures can be complex and sometimes unpredictable. Simple connective tissue grafts or free gingival grafts however can transform recipient sites to improve the appearance and masticatory function of an edentulous saddle. The palate and tuberosity are usually good donor sites for harvesting tissue, as the vascular supply promotes good post-operative healing. Preparation of the recipient site with a vascular bed, immobilisation and wound protection are prerequisites for predictable success. Free gingival grafts are often used to increase the attached width of gingiva, although there may be a colour mismatch.

Recontouring and Regeneration Techniques

Recontouring of the gingival tissues can facilitate periodontal health and improve appearance in those suffering from drug-induced gingival hyperplasia. Osseous recontouring with apically repositioned flaps (chapter 8) can increase the clinical crown height of restorations, based on the concept of biological width.

Various techniques are available to improve the soft tissues associated with fixed prosthodontic restorations and to recreate the interdental papilla – an example being the Palacci technique, developed to regenerate the gingival papilla between implants. This involves cutting semilunar bevel incisions in a straight line buccal flap and rotating the pedicles created to fill the inter-implant/dental spaces.

Conclusions

- Planning for tooth replacement should take place before tooth removal.
- The advent of reliable dental implants has changed the rationale and scope of 'preprosthetic surgery'.
- A number of surgical procedures can be used to modify the hard and soft tissues to facilitate the provision of prostheses and enhance restorative clinical outcomes.
- Practitioners undertaking implant surgery require clinical expertise in minor oral surgery and advanced restorative techniques.

Further Reading

Hobkirk JA, Watson RM. A Colour Atlas and Text of Dental and Maxillofacial Implantology. St Louis: Mosby, 1995.

Hopkins R, Crompton P. A Colour Atlas of Preprosthetic Oral Surgery. St Louis: Mosby, 1990.

Weinberg LA. Atlas of Tooth and Implant Supported Prosthodontics. London: Quintessence Publishing Co Ltd, 2003.

Worthington P, Brånemark P-I (eds). Advanced Osseointegration Surgery: Applications in the Maxillofacial Region. London: Quintessence Publishing Co Ltd, 1993.

Chapter 10
Minor Oral Surgery and the Antrum

Aim

The aim of this chapter is to discuss the ways in which the maxillary antrum can be involved in the practice of minor oral surgery.

Outcome

After reading this chapter you should understand the techniques used to manage oro-antral communications.

Introduction

The antrum may become involved in the surgical treatment of the dentition in a number of ways. During tooth extraction an oro-antral communication (OAC) may be created. This may become epithelialised to form an oro-antral fistula (OAF). A root may be displaced into the antrum or the maxillary tuberosity may fracture. Closure of the antral defect may become necessary either immediately or later. The antrum may be involved in benign pathology such as cysts or be the site of a malignancy. The antrum is frequently involved in maxillofacial trauma and in infection, which may cause difficulty in diagnosis. Finally, prior to the placement of implants, bone grafting of the maxillary sinus floor may be required.

Anatomy
The maxillary antrum has been described as having:
- a pyramidal shape
- four walls
- a floor – which is closely associated with the roots of the upper premolar and molar teeth
- a roof – which is also the floor of the orbit
- a respiratory epithelium lining – which is continuous with the nasal mucosa via the ostium.

Development

The antrum increases in size during childhood and continues to pneumatise with age.

Function

The maxillary antrum has a number of functions. These aid:

- respiration – inspired air is warmed and humidified by circulation over the respiratory mucosa
- speech – the paranasal air spaces of which the antrum is one, give resonation of speech
- lightening of the skull – the weight of the head is limited by the presence of the air cells. This maxillary antrum may also help form a 'crumple zone' to absorb impact in maxillofacial trauma.

Drainage

It is important to appreciate the drainage pattern of the maxillary sinus. The antrum drains into the nose via the ostium, which is approximately half way up the medial wall. The ostium opens into the nose at the level of the middle meatus. Importantly the ciliated mucosa of the lining is extremely efficient and will normally move mucus from the base of the antrum to the ostium in around one hour. Thus drainage is away from the floor and not dependent upon gravity.

Surgical Involvement of the Antrum

The ways in which the antrum can impact on dental practice are described below.

Iatrogenic Injury

There are a number of occasions when the antrum can be involved during oral surgical procedures:

During extraction

This is the most likely way in which the dentist will encounter the antrum. The root apices of the upper teeth are closely associated with this structure. The maxillary sinus may extend as far forward as the upper canine (Fig 10-1). Any extractions in this area may cause a communication between the antrum and the mouth. The root most commonly associated is the palatal

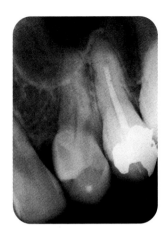

Fig 10-1 The antrum may extend anteriorly beyond the premolar teeth.

root of the upper first permanent molar. This is especially the case when there is evidence of apical pathology, which may cause resorption of the bone of the antral floor. The initial diagnosis is by suspicion (Table 10-1). Where there is any evidence to alert the clinician, the patient must be warned of the possibility of a communication and fistula formation. A conservative regimen may be started to allow healing to take place naturally (Table 10-2).

Patients should be warned not to increase antral pressure by blowing their nose and avoid sneezing. Such actions may cause a communication and possibly a prolapse of the antral lining (Fig 10-2). If the antral lining prolapses,

Table 10-1

INITIAL DIAGNOSIS OF ORO-ANTRAL COMMUNICATION (IMMEDIATELY AFTER EXTRACTION)
NOT BY FORCED NASAL EXPIRATION
NOT BY PROBING
OBSERVATION
SUSPICION
RADIOGRAPH

Table 10-2

CONSERVATIVE REGIMEN TO MANAGE AN ANTRAL COMMUNICATION
PATIENT INSTRUCTIONS – NO NOSE-BLOWING, ORAL HYGEINE INSTRUCTION, etc.
+/-
NASAL DECONGESTANTS – EPHEDRINE 0.5%
+/-
ANTIBIOTICS – BROAD SPECTRUM
REVIEW – UNTIL HEALED

it is unlikely to be easily reduced back into the antrum and will have to be excised. A buccal advanced flap is used to close the defect (see below).

Oro-Antral Communication

An oro-antral communication may occur more frequently than one realises. The condition may remain asymptomatic and heal spontaneously if the communication is not allowed to epithelialise. Initial healing of the socket can be promoted by the use of the conservative regimen described above. A more active protocol (Table 10-3) may involve suturing and packing the socket, together with the use of a splint to stop the reflux of fluids. The socket may be packed with a bioresorbable material such as oxidized cellulose, which will help to stabilise the clot. The defect should never be packed with non-resorbable material such as ribbon gauze, as this will encourage the formation of a permanent fistula.

Splints can be constructed to seal the communication and allow spontaneous healing to take place. These can take the form of an extension to a denture, a soft splint or a hard base-plate (Fig 10-3). Care should be taken to ensure that impression material does not enter the defect, which should be covered with a piece of foil or gauze. Once fitted, the communication between mouth and sinus will be interrupted and this may allow spontaneous healing to take place (Fig 10-3). At the least, it should reduce the chance of infection and give the clinician time to plan a definitive closure.

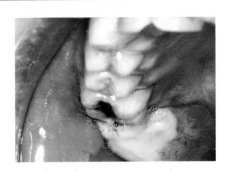

Fig 10-2 Antral prolapse following removal of upper third molar. The patient reported blowing his nose on the evening following extraction.

Table 10-3

ACTIVE REGIMEN TO CLOSE AN ORO-ANTRAL COMMUNICATION
SUTURING
+/-
PACKS
+/-
SPLINTS
+
CONSERVATIVE REGIMEN

Oro-Antral Fistula

An oro-antral fistula may present as a late complication of a communication. There may be symptoms of sinusitis or reflux of fluids from the mouth through the nose (Table 10-4).

In this situation an immediate closure may be delayed until the acute infection has settled. A splint will stop the reflux and may prevent further infection. In some circumstances this has allowed healing of the fistula to occur when surgical intervention has been postponed. Antibiotics may be neces-

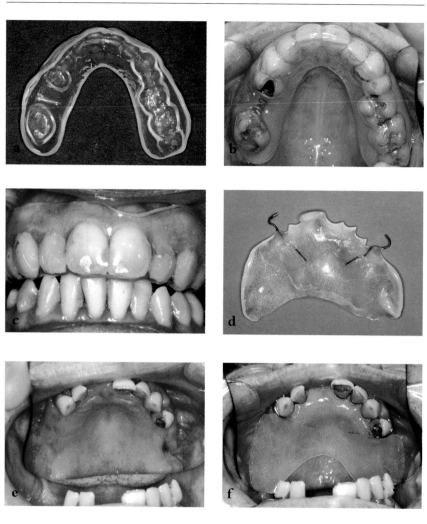

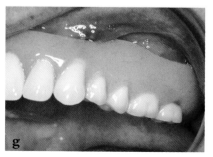

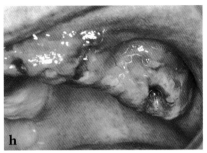
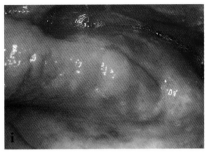

Fig 10-3 Different splints used to seal oro-antral communications. (a) A soft occlusal coverage splint. (b, (c) Soft splint in place. (d) A hard acrylic splint. (e) The oro-antral communication to be covered is obvious. (f) The hard splint in place covering the communication. (g) Denture used to cover an oro-antral communication. (h) The oro-antral communication to be covered is obvious. (i) The healed communication.

sary at the time of closure, which is effected by the use of a buccally advanced mucoperiosteal flap (see below). A three-sided flap should be raised and the fistula track excised to allow connective tissue healing to occur. In addition, a conservative regimen as outlined above is of value.

Immediate Retrieval of a Root From the Antrum
Apical fragments can easily be dislodged into the antrum and will need to be retrieved. A radiograph (a pantomogram, occipitomental, oblique occlusal or periapical views) may be taken to identify the position of the root (Fig 10-4) and a decision made as to the best way of proceeding. The root can be removed immediately through the tooth socket after raising a three-sided mucoperiosteal flap (Fig 10-5). Bone is then removed to improve access and vision and the root can often either be seen directly or removed with powerful suction.

Table 10-4

LATE DIAGNOSIS OF AN ORO-ANTRAL FISTULA
REFLUX OF FLUID, SMOKE, etc. INTO NOSE
REFLUX OF FLUID INTO MOUTH
DISCHARGE, BAD TASTE
SINUSITIS

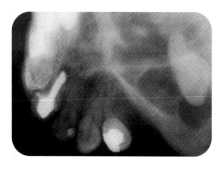

Fig 10-4 A radiograph showing the presence of a tooth in the antrum.

Buccally Advanced Flap

Oro-antral communications may be closed by advancing a mucoperiosteal flap. A three-sided flap is raised on the buccal side of the defect (Fig 10-5b). This will not stretch across to the palatal aspect of the communication due to the inelastic nature of the periosteal layer of the flap. This is overcome by incising the periosteum alone at the level of the reflection (Fig 10-5c). This allows the more elastic connective tissue to stretch enabling the flap to be sutured to the palatal mucosa without tension (Fig 10-5d, g). The intention is to cover the defect with an island of mucoperiosteum, which will encourage new bone formation. The flap is sutured in place with its margins over sound bone with particular emphasis on the palatal edge (sacrifice of the fistula lining should be extended to produce a shelf of bone on the palatal aspect (Fig 10-5e,f)). Single interrupted or mattress sutures can be employed (Fig 10-5g) but the flap will require support for up to two weeks. Once an airtight seal has been achieved the ciliated lining mucosa of the sinus will re-establish an efficient drainage pattern.

Palatal Rotation Flap

This technique is described in many texts but is infrequently used for the closure of oro-antral defects. Its principal use is in the closure of oro-nasal fistulae that present in the palate or when it is impossible to advance a buccal flap. An example of the latter is when a communication is produced following removal of a palatally placed upper premolar and the teeth in the line of the arch have tight contact points.

The flap design, based on the greater palatine vessels, is shown in Fig 10-6. The palatal flap may be considered if buccal advancement flaps have failed. They have the advantage of maintaining sulcus depth. The disadvantages of the palatal flap include exposure of bone and fluid leakage at the palatal aspect, as it is difficult to compress the flap against bone at this point.

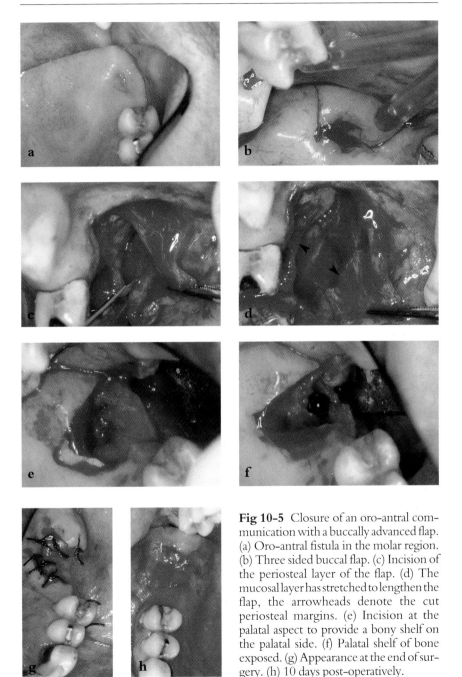

Fig 10-5 Closure of an oro-antral communication with a buccally advanced flap. (a) Oro-antral fistula in the molar region. (b) Three sided buccal flap. (c) Incision of the periosteal layer of the flap. (d) The mucosal layer has stretched to lengthen the flap, the arrowheads denote the cut periosteal margins. (e) Incision at the palatal aspect to provide a bony shelf on the palatal side. (f) Palatal shelf of bone exposed. (g) Appearance at the end of surgery. (h) 10 days post-operatively.

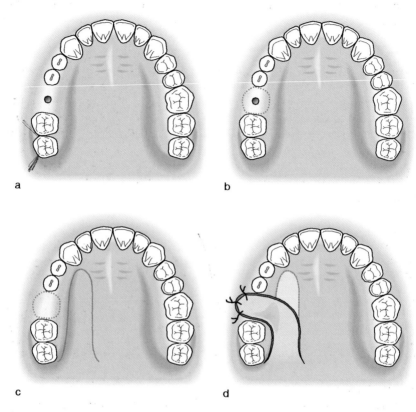

Fig 10-6 The design of the palatal flap to close oro-antral communications. (a) position of the communication in the first molar region. (b) margin of communication excised. (c) palatal flap outlined. (d) palatal flap rotated over communication and sutured in place leaving defect in the anterior palate.

Delayed Removal of the Root

If removal of a root displaced into the antrum is delayed, the socket may heal spontaneously and the clinician may choose to retrieve the root using a Caldwell-Luc approach. This is achieved by raising a buccal mucoperiosteal flap in the premolar and canine sulcus region. The incision should be placed supragingivally. Bone is then removed over the apices of the teeth to gain access to the sinus. The root may be difficult to visualise, as it can move into one of the convolutions of the sinus. Irrigation of the sinus may be necessary to dislodge the root, at which time it can be retrieved using suction. The wound should be closed to ensure an airtight seal and the patient should be placed on antibiotics and nasal decongestants.

Fractured Tuberosity
This is a complication of extraction of upper molar teeth, particularly those which are lone-standing and unopposed (see Chapter 5). The incidence increases with loss of bone elasticity, and care should be taken in these circumstances to reduce the support of the tooth by using Couplands elevators (see Chapter 5) or adopting a surgical approach. If the tuberosity is felt to fracture then a flap should be raised and the extraction completed by freeing the tooth from the bone using a bur. A large defect into the antrum may be created, and this will have to be closed using the buccal advancement technique described above.

Infection
Infection of an upper tooth may spread through the thin apical bone and involve the antrum directly. Alternatively, infection of the antrum may give rise to symptoms of apical pathology. Appropriate vitality tests and radiographs can help clarify this diagnostic difficulty. After correction of an oroantral fistula symptoms of sinusitis may persist despite apparently good closure. This is probably due to alteration of the activity of the respiratory mucosa and reduced drainage from the ostium. Referral to an ear, nose and throat surgeon should be considered in these cases.

Implant Surgery
Prior to placement of implants the antral floor needs to be surveyed to ensure that sufficient bone is present. Sinus augmentation procedures were described in Chapter 9.

Trauma
The antrum is frequently involved in trauma to the mid-third of the face, in particular fractures of the zygomatic bone. Fractures in this area will cause haemorrhage into the antrum, which may present as an epistaxis. Radiographs will show opacity of the antrum or a fluid level (Fig 10-7). Blowing of the nose can cause surgical emphysema. Patients, even those with an undisplaced fracture, should be warned not to increase intra-antral pressure.

Cysts
Cysts associated with the upper teeth can involve the antrum as they enlarge. In the early stages the cyst cavity is usually separate from the

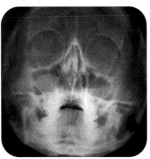

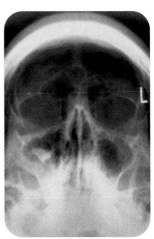

Fig 10-7 Fracture left zygoma with a fluid level apparent in the left antrum; a symptomless mucocele is present on the right side.

Fig 10-8 A keratocyst in the antrum, it has displaced the upper third molar into the maxillary sinus.

antrum, but infection may cause a communication and the removal of the cyst may necessitate careful repair to avoid an oro-antral fistula. Dentigerous cysts associated with upper third molars, premolars or canine teeth can also involve the antrum. Similarly, keratocysts may involve the antrum (Fig 10-8).

Neoplasia
Involvement of the antrum in neoplastic lesions is relatively rare but can be significant. This is especially the case with malignant lesions. The first presentation may be at a late stage in the disease when spread of the tumour is well advanced. Unexplained epistaxis, infra-orbital nerve paraesthesia, loose maxillary teeth, cloudiness of the antrum and loss of bone on radiographs are all signs that should be explored to exclude this diagnosis. Squamous cell carcinoma, adenocarcinoma, sarcoma and lymphoma have all been described arising from the antrum.

Conclusions
- The antrum is an important part of the respiratory system.
- Dentists can encounter the antrum in a number of ways.

- Iatrogenic injury is common particularly associated with the extraction of the first permanent molar.
- Oro-antral communications can be managed conservatively.
- Splints can be useful in the management of oro-antral communications.
- The buccal advanced flap is the usual technique for surgical closure of defects.
- Tumours should be suspected with unexplained antral symptoms.

Further Reading

Anavi Y, Gal G, Silfen R, Calderon S. Palatal rotation–advancement flap for delayed repair of oroantral fistula: a retrospective evaluation of 63 cases. Oral Surg Oral Med Oral Pathol Oral Radiol Endod 2003;96:527-34.

McGowan DA, Baxter PW, James J. The Maxillary Sinus and its Dental Implications. Oxford: Wright, 1993.

Chapter 11
Management of Cysts

Aim

This chapter describes the management of cysts of the mouth and jaws.

Outcome

After reading this chapter you should have an understanding of the techniques used to treat cysts affecting the oral structures.

Introduction

Cysts are pathological cavities containing fluid, semi-fluid or gaseous contents. They do not contain pus unless secondarily infected. They are usually epithelial-lined but the solitary (traumatic) bone cyst and aneurysmal bone cysts are exceptions to this. The radicular cyst (associated with the apex of a non-vital tooth) is the commonest odontogenic cyst. Cysts are not neoplastic. Very rarely malignant change may occur.

How do Cysts Form?

There are several theories of cyst formation. One of these suggests proliferation of the epithelial lining due to some unknown stimulus. Another theory suggests accumulation of fluid in the cyst as a result of hydrostatic forces resulting in resorption of any surrounding bone. Bony resorption is integral to facilitating cyst enlargement when the cyst lies within bone.

Clinical Presentation (Table 11-1)

Dental cysts are often asymptomatic and are noted as incidental radiographic findings. Others may produce signs and symptoms. Any infected cyst may present with pain and swelling, much like an abscess.

Swelling may occur in the absence of infection (Fig 11-1). If enough bony resorption has occurred, an 'eggshell' layer of overlying subperiosteal new bone is present, which will often be felt to crack on palpation. Depending

Table 11-1

Presentation of cysts
INCIDENTAL FINDING ON A RADIOGRAPH
SWELLING
BONY EXPANSION
INFECTION (PAIN AND SWELLING)
DISPLACEMENT/LOOSENING OF TEETH/DENTURE
ALTERED SENSATION

on the position of the cyst, displacement or loosening of teeth may occur. An enlarging cyst may cause problems in relation to the fit of a denture.

Altered sensation may be produced by pressure on anatomically related nerves. The latter is less common than might be expected, given the relatively slow speed of cyst enlargement. A rapid increase in size may occur if the cyst is infected. Altered sensation is a symptom that should always be taken seriously, as it may imply neoplasia.

Occasionally, a large cyst may cause a pathological fracture of the mandible. Cysts of the minor salivary glands (Fig 11-2) occur on the lip vermillion, cheeks, floor of mouth and palate. The cause is often trauma (e.g. lip or cheek biting). Saliva can then accumulate subsequent to duct rupture or stenosis. The two types recognised are mucous retention and mucous extravasation cysts. These are most common in children and adolescents. The cysts usually present as smooth fluid-containing bluish swellings. Periodically, they may burst but inevitably reform. In the floor of the mouth cysts arising from the sublingual gland may grow to large sizes and are denoted by the term ranula (Fig 11-3).

Sometimes an ectopic part of the submandibular salivary gland invaginates the bone of the mandible near the angle. This appears as a well-defined corticated radiolucency below the inferior alveolar canal. It is known as a Stafne's bone cavity or cyst but requires no treatment.

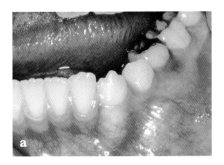

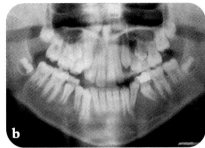

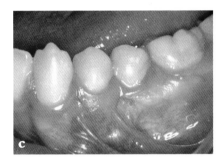

Fig 11-1 A dentigerous cyst associated with an unerupted lower second premolar. (a) Clinical appearance at presentation showing buccal swelling (b) Radiographic appearance at presentation. (c) Clinical appearance after treatment by marsupialisation showing erupted lower second premolar.

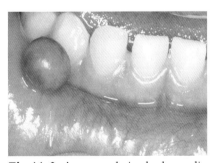

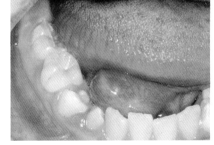

Fig 11-2 A mucocele in the lower lip of a three-year-old child.

Fig 11-3 A ranula.

Investigations

History and clinical examination are important. Radiographic examination is also essential to determine the site and extent of intrabony lesions. Often two views at different angles are useful to examine for expansion of bone (Fig 11-4), which may also be evident clinically. Well-corticated margins

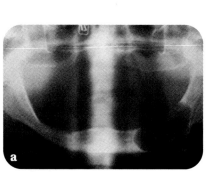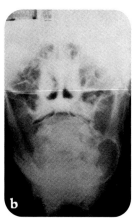

Fig 11-4 Radiographs showing a large residual cyst in the mandible. (a) A dental panoramic view. (b) A posterior-anterior mandibular view.

are usually seen, but these often become indistinct when there is a history of infection.

Electric pulp-testing of teeth close to the cyst can provide valuable information as to the etiology. Teeth with radicular cysts (see below) are non-vital.

In modern practice, aspiration is often not carried out initially. It may be carried out immediately prior to surgery, if there is doubt about the nature of the lesion. When managing more extensive lesions, a biopsy (see Chapter 13) should be taken of the cyst lining prior to more definitive surgery, once the nature of the lesion has been elucidated. An aspirate containing less than 40g per litre of soluble protein suggests an odontogenic keratocyst.

Classification

There are several classifications of cysts, but the World Health Organization (WHO) classification, which was revised in 1992, is often used. It is important to have an idea of cyst derivation as it may affect aspects of treatment (Table 11-2).

Odontogenic Cysts
Odontogenic keratocyst
These cysts lie in the tooth-bearing regions of the jaws or distal to the mandibular third molars (Fig 11-5). They originate from the dental lamina.

Table 11-2 **The WHO classification of cysts (1992)**

EPITHELIAL CYSTS	AGE AT PRESENTATION (Decade)
Developmental	
Odontogenic	
Keratocyst	2,3
Dentigerous cyst	3,4
Lateral periodontal cyst	variable
Eruption cyst	1,2
Gingival cyst	1
Non-odontogenic	
Nasopalatine duct cyst	4,5,6
Nasolabial cyst	4,5
Inflammatory	
Radicular (apical, lateral, residual)	4,5
Paradental cyst	variable

NON-EPITHELIAL PSEUDOCYST	
Aneurysmal bone cyst	2
Solitary bone cyst	2

These cysts are more common in men than women and appear radiographically as multilocular radiolucencies in most cases. Recurrence after enucleation (see later) is not uncommon, and thus long-term follow-up of these patients is required. The presence of satellite cysts is the main reason for this risk of recurrence. Some authorities recommend the use of Carnoy's solution, which fixes the cyst lining prior to its removal. Others apply cryotherapy to the resultant bony defect after enucleation.

Histologically, as well as satellite cysts a capsule lined with parakeratinised stratified squamous epithelium is seen. The epithelium is usually of an even thickness (around five to 10 cells).

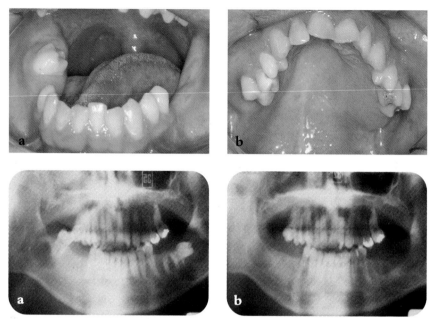

Fig 11-5 Multiple keratocysts in a patient with Gorlin-Goltz syndrome. (a) Swellings in both lower molar regions are apparent. (b) Swelling is visible in the upper left molar region. (c) Radiographic appearance showing radiolucencies in the upper left and both lower molar regions. (d) Radiographic appearance showing healing after treatment of the multiple cysts by enucleation.

Multiple keratocysts may occur as part of the Gorlin-Goltz syndrome (Fig 11-5) in which multiple basal cell skin cancers are also seen, together with bifid ribs, abnormalities of the vertebrae and intracranial abnormalities (e.g. calcification of the falx cerebri). In this syndrome there are characteristic facies with frontal and parietal bossing and a broad nasal root.

Dentigerous (follicular) cysts
These cysts are suspected radiographically when the cyst-like lesion encloses the crown of an unerupted tooth (Figs 11-1 and 11-6). As well as occurring around the crowns of the normal dentition, they can be associated with supernumeraries (Fig 11-7) and odontomes. They are more common in men and develop when fluid accumulates between the crown and reduced enamel epithelium, or within the reduced enamel epithelium itself. Treatment is by removal of the cyst along with the impacted tooth or marsupialisation if the tooth can reach a functional position (Figs 11-1c).

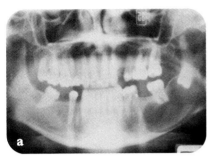 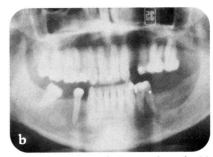

Fig 11-6 A dentigerous cyst treated by enucleation and loss of associated tooth. (a) Radiographic appearance at presentation showing a large dentigerous cyst associated with an unerupted lower left third molar tooth. (b) Radiographic appearance after treatment of cyst by enucleation and loss of the unerupted lower third and erupted lower second molars.

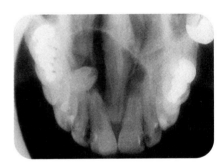

Fig 11-7 A dentigerous cyst associated with a supernumerary tooth in the maxilla.

Histologically the layers of epithelium are cuboidal or squamous in nature.

Lateral periodontal cysts
These cysts are most common in the mandibular premolar region. They occur lateral to or between tooth roots. They are often incidental findings on radiographs. They should be treated by enucleation.

Eruption cysts
These follicular cysts lie partly outside bone and surround the crowns of erupting teeth (Fig 11-8). The lining is of stratified squamous epithelium. Clinically a bluish swelling is seen on the alveolar crest overlying the area of a tooth that is about to erupt. Occasionally excision may be performed, but usually these cysts are treated conservatively, since they resolve when the tooth erupts.

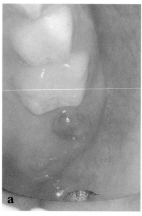
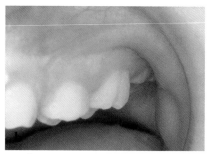

Fig 11-8 An eruption cyst in the upper first permanent molar region. (a) Clinical appearance of the eruption cyst. (b) Eruption of tooth occurred spontaneously one week after Fig 11-8a was taken.

Gingival cysts

These are found in neonates but are rare after three months of age. Many undergo spontaneous resolution. Keratinised nodules on the gingivae are referred as Bohn's Nodules or Epstein's Pearls. No treatment is required.

Non–odontogenic Cysts

Nasopalatine duct cysts

These cysts arise from epithelial remnants in the nasopalatine canal in the midline of the anterior maxilla. They are more commonly seen in men than women. A radiolucent lesion is seen between the upper central incisors. Obviously the nasopalatine canal is a normal radiolucency in this zone. When the radiolucency is more than 10mm in diameter, a cyst should be suspected. Nasopalatine duct cysts are treated by enucleation. They are lined with a layer of pseudostratified ciliated columnar epithelium.

Nasolabial cysts

This cyst is found on the alveolar process near the base of the nostril and is entirely contained within soft tissue. There are therefore no radiological signs. They are thought to arise from the lower end of the nasolacrimal duct and are more common in women. These cysts are treated by enucleation. They are lined by non–ciliated pseudostratified columnar epithelium.

Dermoid cysts

These cysts arise from the inclusion of ectoderm at sites of fusion and may occur anywhere in the body. In the mouth they can be found in the palate, the tongue or the floor. They are lined by stratified squamous epithelium and are treated by enucleation.

When arising in the floor of the mouth they may be found in the midline or laterally but do not become obvious until adolescence or adulthood. Clinical examination shows a fluctuant or soft swelling that may lie above or below the mylohyoid muscle. It does not move up or down on swallowing (unlike a thyroglossal cyst).

Inflammatory Cysts
Radicular cysts
These arise from the epithelial rest cells of Malassez in the periodontal ligament. They are stimulated to proliferate by inflammation following pulpal death and may be apical or lateral in position. They are more common in men and appear as unilocular well-defined oval or round radiolucencies, but the margins are less well-defined in infected cases. The radiographic appearance can be similar to that of an apical granuloma, but lesions with a diameter exceeding 10mm are more likely to be cystic. Radicular cysts should be enucleated.

If the cyst remains after a tooth has been removed it is known as a residual cyst. These lesions may resolve without treatment; if they persist they should be enucleated.

Paradental cysts
These occur as a result of inflammation occurring in a periodontal pocket. They are often associated with an unerupted third molar. The cysts are attached to the enamel-cement junction and are treated by enucleation.

Non-Epithelial Entities
Aneurysmal bone cysts (ABC)
This intra-osseous lesion, seen mainly in the mandible, consists of blood-filled spaces. It also contains fibroblastic tissue and multinucleated giant cells, osteoid and woven bone. Slightly more common in women, aneurysmal bone cysts are seen mostly in the first and second decades. Radiographically, the characteristic feature is of multiloccular radiolucency. Surgical excision is recommended as treatment, but since there may be much haemorrhage, patients with this lesion should be managed in hospital.

Solitary (traumatic, simple, haemorrhagic) bone cysts
These lesions do not have an epithelial lining. They are lined by fibrovas-

cular connective tissue. They are most commonly seen in the second decade of life and often have no fluid content. Radiographically they appear as a well-defined radiolucency. The roots of neighbouring teeth may be displaced. After exploration spontaneous involution of the cyst usually occurs. Aspiration of air confirms the diagnosis, and no further investigation is necessary.

Surgical Management

The mainstays of surgical treatment of cysts are:
* enucleation
* marsupialisation.

Enucleation of a cyst is the technique of choice in most circumstances. It involves complete removal of the cyst and primary closure of overlying soft tissue. An example of enucleation is where a cyst is removed from the apical region of a tooth at the time of apicectomy (see Chapter 7).

In some cases it may be necessary to perform marsupialisation. Such treatment occurs where complete removal may cause unacceptable disruption to the surrounding anatomy. Examples of this include cases where enucleation might result in damage to the inferior alveolar nerve in the mandible, the mandible itself (Fig 11-4) or involvement of the floor of the nose or maxillary antrum. This technique is also used when managing a dentigerous cyst associated with an unerupted tooth that is to be maintained (Fig 11-1). The idea behind this type of treatment is that the defect will gradually shrink, allowing possible enucleation at a later date. In some cases involution of the lesion may render subsequent treatment unnecessary.

Treatment Technique
Enucleation (Fig 11-9)
This may be performed under local or general anaesthesia, depending on the extent of the lesion. When designing the soft tissue flap, it is important wherever possible to ensure that the incision line does not lie over the surgical defect. The thinned bone should be removed over the cyst using either a bur or rongeurs. As far as possible, using a curette, the cyst lining should be peeled away from the bony cavity. It is sometimes helpful to do this using half-inch ribbon gauze held in some forceps and pushing away the cyst lining from the bone by placing the gauze between the two layers.

After the cyst has been removed it is sent in 10% neutral buffered formalin for

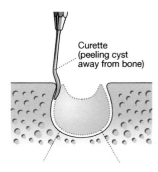

Fig 11-9 The technique of cyst enucleation.

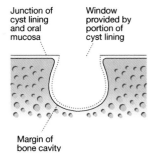

Fig 11-10 The technique of cyst marsupialisation.

histopathological examination (see Chapter 13). The resultant bony defect is closed primarily, and there is no need for packing of the cyst cavity.

Marsupialisation (Fig 11-10)
In this technique, the cyst is opened and a window of cyst lining and overlying soft tissue is removed with it. The cyst cavity is drained and the margin of the window where the cyst lining and epithelium meet can be sutured. The resultant cavity can be packed with ribbon gauze impregnated with Bismuth Iodoform Paraffin Paste (BIPP) or Whitehead's varnish. Such packs are removed initially at weekly intervals and gradually reduced in size as the cavity becomes smaller. In some situations dentures have been constructed with a bung filling the surgical cavity. The bung is periodically reduced in size as the defect reduces. This approach can be a little laborious and, of course, requires the additional services of a technician. A disadvantage of marsupialisation is that only a part of the lining is available for histopathological examination.

Conclusions

Cysts, which can present in various forms in the mouth, can be treated by enucleation or marsupialisation.

Further Reading

Cawson RA, Binnie WH, Eveson JW. Colour Atlas of Oral Disease. 2nd edn. London: Mosby-Wolfe, 1994.

Cawson RA, Langdon JD, Eveson JW. Surgical Pathology of the Mouth and Jaws. Oxford: Wright, 1996.

Moore UJ (ed). Principles of Oral and Maxillofacial Surgery. 5th edn. Oxford: Blackwell Science, 2001.

Chapter 12
Management of Dento-alveolar Trauma and Oral Lacerations

Aim

This chapter describes the management of trauma to the hard and soft tissues of the mouth.

Outcome

After reading this chapter you should have an understanding of the techniques used to treat dental and oral soft-tissue injuries.

Introduction

The incidence of dento-alveolar trauma is higher in children than adults (Fig 12-1). In all cases it is important in the first instance to remember that other, more serious injuries may be associated. It is therefore important to bear in mind the principles of ATLS (Advanced Trauma Life Support), which underpin the management of all cases of trauma.

Primary Survey

The degree to which this is carried out will depend on the overall appearance of the patient at presentation. The primary survey may have been performed before the patient attends the dental surgery. The same principles should be borne in mind for all patients. They are given in Table 12-1. The

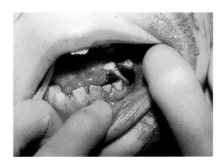

Fig 12-1 A dento-alveolar fracture in a child.

Table 12-1 **Features of the primary survey – identification and management of life-threatening injures**

Primary Survey
AIRWAY MAINTENANCE – CERVICAL SPINE CONTROL (UNCONSCIOUS = UNABLE TO MAINTAIN OWN AIRWAY)
BREATHING
CIRCULATION – AND CONTROL OF HAEMORRHAGE
DISABILITY – NEUROLOGICAL DEFICIT (GLASGOW COMA SCALE – BASED ON GRADED RESPONSES TO MOTOR, VERBAL AND VISUAL STIMULI)
EXPOSURE – TO LOOK FOR OTHER INJURIES (AND ENVIRON-MENTAL CONTROL)

most pertinent example of this is a patient presenting with dento-alveolar injury who gives a history of loss of consciousness. If such an event is not considered fully then potential danger can arise. The Glasgow Coma Scale (Table 12-2) is a useful tool in assessing the degree of head injury and is helpful in describing the patient when referring on for further management.

Secondary Survey

This is carried out once the patient's general condition is stabilised and entails a detailed head-to-toe examination. In the dental surgery, the secondary survey may be covered by relevant questions in the history if the trauma has been relatively minor and the primary survey has yielded nothing. It is at this point that radiographs appropriate to the injury or suspected injury should be carried out.

Points in the History

In the conscious patient, a thorough history must be obtained. This should include details of when, where and how the incident happened (particularly in cases of alleged assault) and the mechanism of injury. The latter may give

Table 12-2 **Glasgow Coma Scale (GCS) - measures motor responsiveness, verbal performance, eye opening**

Motor responsiveness scores (GCS)

6 = obeys commands   ☐
5 = localises pain   ☐
4 = withdraws from pain   ☐
3 = flexor response to pain   ☐
2 = extensor response to pain   ☐
1 = no response to pain   ☐

Best verbal performance scores (GCS)

5 = orientated   ☐
4 = confused conversation   ☐
3 = inappropriate speech   ☐
2 = incomprehensible speech   ☐
1 = no response   ☐

Eye-opening scores (GCS)

4 = spontaneous   ☐
3 = to speech   ☐
2 = to pain   ☐
1 = none   ☐

GCS score <8 = severe injury
GCS score 9-12 = moderate injury
GCS score 13-15 = minor injury

a clue as to associated injuries that may be present. From what has been said previously, it is clear that the patient should be asked whether or not they lost consciousness. If the answer is yes then the patient should be asked the last thing they remember and what was the first thing they remembered after regaining consciousness. This may indicate the duration of loss of con-

Table 12-3 **Points on a 'Head Injury Card' which should prompt a patient to return to hospital**

Head Injury Card
NAUSEA/VOMITING
INCREASING LETHARGY
INCREASING HEADACHE
VISUAL DISTURBANCES

sciousness. Other clues to this include statements from witnesses. Any patient who gives a history suggestive of loss of consciousness should be transferred to hospital, with an escort. If they are not admitted they will be given an information card advising them to return to hospital if any symptoms such as those shown in Table 12-3 appear.

Dental Injuries

As stated previously, these are more common in children. It is important that non-accidental injury is borne in mind. Features suggestive of non-accidental injury include delayed presentation and injuries that do not appear to be consistent with the suggested mechanism. Multiple injuries, particularly those that appear to be of different ages, are also a cause for concern. Local area Child Protection Committee Guidelines will be available to aid the dental practitioner in their referral. A particular intra-oral sign, which should be sought, is the torn fraenal attachment.

The reader is referred to texts on restorative dentistry for the management of the different types of dental injury.

Dento-Alveolar Fractures

Dento-alveolar fractures constitute fractures of the tooth-bearing part of the mandible/maxilla (Fig 12-1).

Wires, bars and acrylic splints may all find applications in the treatment of dento-alveolar fractures. Bars (Fig 12-2) and splints are usually constructed in the den-

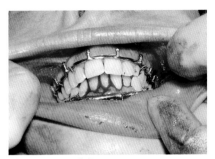

Fig 12-2 Arch bars.

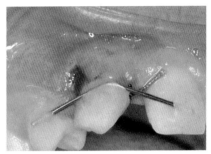

Fig 12-3 An acid-etch composite and wire splint used to support a mobile tooth.

tal laboratory on initial impressions. An increasing number of practitioners are now using acid-etch retained composite splints (Fig 12-3) and orthodontic bands in these situations. At least four weeks' splinting is required.

In some cases it is possible to stabilise a dento-alveolar fracture using mini-plates in the same manner as they are used to treat a fractured mandible. The bony fragment is stabilised by adapting plates across the fracture site, ensuring that two screws are inserted on either side of the fracture to eliminate rotation. It is unlikely that this equipment will be available in dental practice. Thus, if this treatment is needed, referral to a specialist oral and maxillofacial unit is appropriate.

All of the devices depend on the splint joining the injured, mobile segment to the uninjured stable segment.

Oral Lacerations

As with all injuries, a thorough history should be obtained. Oral lacerations either occur as a result of injury or in some cases iatrogenic damage.

Examination should obtain the site and extent of injury. Extent includes depth of the injury as well as its surface appearance. The former is particularly significant, as there may be damage to important underlying structures. These are summarised in Table 12-4.

Radiographs

These should be taken when there may be root fractures, an underlying bony injury or the presence of a foreign body is suspected. It should be remem-

Table 12-4

Anatomical structures to be remembered in intra-oral lacerations
PAROTID DUCT
SUBMANDIBULAR DUCT
LINGUAL NERVE
LINGUAL ARTERY
MENTAL NERVE
FACIAL NERVE
FACIAL ARTERY

bered that not all foreign bodies are radiopaque, and therefore the wound should be thoroughly debrided and examined prior to closure to exclude presence. Soft-tissue radiographic examinations that have a decreased exposure are useful (Fig 12-4).

Treatment of Lacerations

Lacerations involving the vermillion border of the lips are injuries that need care when closing. A mismatch of the junction between the skin and vermillion can be particularly obvious after healing has occurred. If the laceration is deep, underlying resorbable sutures are required prior to placing the surface sutures. The underlying sutures should be undyed. A fine monofilament suture such as 5/0 nylon should be used on the skin and vermillion surfaces.

In terms of intra-oral lacerations, it is surprising how many of these will heal spontaneously, provided they are not contaminated. Consideration should always be given to managing these injuries conservatively. Examples are injuries that occur to the tongue. These are often seen in children and frequently heal without operative treatment. If the laceration involves the lateral border of the tongue then it is more likely that suturing will be required. Tongue injuries that repeatedly bleed or are at risk of extensive bleeding should always be considered for closure. This is particularly important in

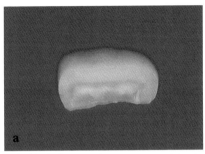
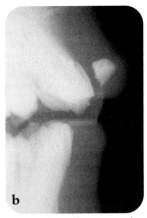

Fig 12-4 (a) A fractured upper central incisor tip. (b) The soft tissue radiograph showing the dental remnant in the lip.

children due to their low circulating blood volume. A resorbable suture such as 3/0 or 4/0 vicryl should be used in such circumstances.

Most intra-oral lacerations may be managed using local anaesthesia and are suitably treated in the dental surgery. Exceptions to this include inaccessible areas (e.g. the soft palate or fauces), but many of these cases will heal well without suturing.

Skin Lacerations
These are usually (unless very superficial) closed in layers. The deep layer is closed with a material such as vicryl, which is resorbable. The 4/0 size should be used, and in the case of skin lacerations the undyed variety should be chosen. The surface sutures are usually unresorbable and removed after five days. They comprise materials such as ethilon or prolene. A narrow gauge suture such as 5/0 should be used. In the case of small lacerations (e.g. of the lip in children) it is worth considering the use of a material that is resorbable, since removal may require a general anaesthetic. This should only be done if aesthetics are not compromised.

Intra-oral Lacerations
In cases that require suturing vicryl (3/0 or 4/0) should be used. The dyed variety may be used in this situation. Unless a rapidly resorbable variety is used, the sutures often take some weeks to resorb.

Use of Antibiotics

Amoxicillin may be used in the case of intra-oral lacerations. This may be supplemented with metronidazole when the wound is heavily contaminated.

Conclusions

- More serious injuries should be investigated in cases of dental trauma.
- Traumatic injuries to the teeth are managed in a variety of ways.
- Some intra-oral lacerations can be treated conservatively.

Further Reading

Advanced Trauma Life Support Student Manual. Chicago, Illinois: American College of Surgeons, 1997.

Coulthard P, Horner K, Sloan P, Theaker ED. Master Dentistry: Oral and Maxillofacial Surgery, Radiology, Pathology and Oral Medicine. Edinburgh: Churchill Livingstone, 2003.

Williams JL (ed). Rowe and Williams Maxillofacial Injuries. Edinburgh: Churchill Livingstone, 1994.

Chapter 13

Biopsy Techniques and Management of Intra-oral Calculi

Aim

This chapter describes biopsy techniques and the removal of salivary calculi.

Outcome

After reading this chapter you should understand the principles of biopsy and salivary calculus removal.

Biopsy Techniques

Prior to undertaking any form of biopsy a thorough history and examination should be carried out. This may provide a clue as to the nature of the lesion. When dealing with intra-oral lesions special attention should be paid to the smoking and alcohol history, together with details of any parafunctional habits.

A biopsy is a means of providing a specimen of tissue that is then subjected to histopathological examination. These are listed in Table 13-1.

Biopsies may be performed in dental practice. It is important to stress, however, that if a lesion is suspected of being a malignancy the patient should be referred as a matter of urgency to a specialist oral and maxillofacial surgery unit (Fig 13-1). Lesions that appear malignant should not be biopsied in the general practice setting. One reason for this is that the exact location and dimensions of the lesion may not be apparent to the team that is eventually going to treat the patient. The two principal methods of biopsy used in general practice are the incisional and excisional types. Both procedures may be carried out under local anaesthesia. Lesions in inaccessible areas such as the posterior soft palate or back of tongue may require general anaesthesia and thus referral to a specialist unit. When injecting local anaesthetic prior to the biopsy it is important not to inject into the area that is being removed. This is to prevent tissue distortion by the injected solution.

Table 13-1

Biopsy techniques

Excisional biopsy (whole of lesion removed)

Incisional biopsy (part of lesion removed)

Curettings

Punch biopsy

Fine needle aspiration biopsy

Brush biopsy

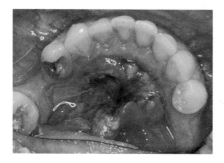

Fig 13-1 This floor of mouth lesion is highly suspicious of a malignancy. Biopsy of such lesions is contraindicated in general dental practice. Urgent referral to a maxillofacial surgeon is the appropriate treatment.

Surgical Techniques

Incisional and excisional biopsies are carried out using sharp dissection so that any crush artefact of the specimen is minimised. Crushing of the specimen may render it useless for a histological diagnosis and necessitate a further surgical procedure for the patient. If instruments such as toothed forceps hold the specimen then these should be used at the periphery of the sample. This avoids crushing the main area of interest. The preferred method of preventing crushing is to use a suture to hold the specimen (Fig 13-2). The suture should be inserted before using the scalpel. The suture can be used to hold the specimen during removal and transfer to the transport container. Another advantage of inserting a suture is that it can be used to orientate the sample. Indeed, for large specimens a suture placed through one

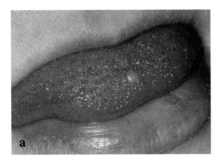
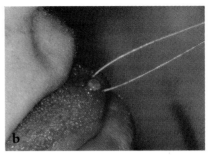
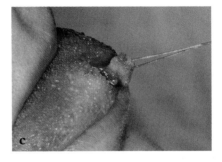

Fig 13-2 Use of a suture to hold a biopsy specimen. (a) The lesion for biopsy on the tip of the tongue. (b) A suture passed below the lesion. (c) The specimen is held by the suture preventing crushing of the sample.

end is recommended. Informing the pathologist of the position of the suture enables orientation. If the suture is lost during transfer this should be mentioned in the pathology request form, as it may confuse diagnosis. The needle should be removed from the end of the suture prior to transfer to the laboratory to avoid needle-stick injury.

In excisional biopsies the whole lesion is removed (Fig 13-3). The technique is suitable for small lesions that appear clinically benign, such as papillomas or polyps. When removing a mucocele (Fig 13-4), any normal minor salivary glands noted in the surgical field should be excised, as these may have been traumatised during the surgery. Any damaged glands that remain may produce a further mucocele. When performing an excisional biopsy, an elliptical incision is normally used. The longer dimension should be parallel to important structures to avoid damage (see below). When excising benign lesions, a 1–2 mm margin of normal tissue is included.

With incisional biopsies, the whole lesion is not removed, but a clinically representative sample is taken in order to facilitate diagnosis and therefore provide a basis for appropriate subsequent treatment (Fig 13-5). Elliptical

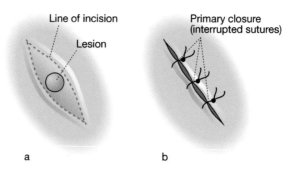

Line of incision

Lesion

Primary closure
(interrupted sutures)

a   b

Fig 13-3 The technique of excisional biopsy.

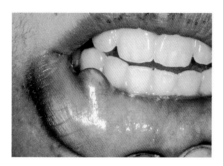

Fig 13-4 When removing mucoceles any surrounding minor salivary glands included in the surgical site should be included.

incisions are recommended. An important factor that determines the position of an incisional biopsy of a large lesion is the position of other important structures. Areas close to the parotid and submandibular ducts and neurovascular bundles such as the mental, lingual and greater palatine nerves should be avoided. Incisional biopsy may be used to diagnosis the nature of mucosal lesions, such as red and white patches. A non-healing ulcer should also be biopsied in this way. A morphologically normal piece of tissue should be removed in continuity with the lesion to show the pathologist the junction between the two. When performing an incisional biopsy in a suspected vesiculo–bullous disorder, it is important not to sample an ulcerated lesion (Fig 13-6). The presence of epithelium is important if immunofluorescent studies are to be performed. Some important principles of biopsy technique are given in Table 13-2.

Given the small size, an incisional biopsy of an intra-oral salivary gland tumour may be difficult to interpret. Therefore, when dealing with well-encapsulated lesions which are small (i.e. not more than 2mm in maximum

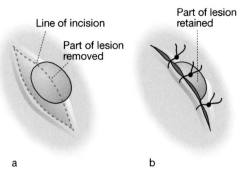

Fig 13-5 The technique of incisonal biopsy.

Table 13-2

Biopsy principles

Do not inject local anaesthetic into the lesion

Biopsy the most suspicious looking area

Include an adequate depth (2mm) to the lesion as well as an adequate surface dimension

The biopsy edge should not bevel inwards as the sample gets deeper

In large lesions more than one area may need to be biopsied

If clinical suspicion persists, even after the report has been obtained in cases of incisional biopsy, the procedure should be repeated

dimension located in the lip, buccal mucosa, tongue and floor of mouth) the taking of an excisional biopsy should be considered, whether there is previous fine needle aspiration biopsy (FNAB – see later) for determination of tissue type or not. In these circumstances the patient should be informed that additional treatment might be needed after the specimen has been subjected to histopathological examination. This may entail further local surgery or radiotherapy.

When dealing with a palatal tumour (which is often well-circumscribed), an

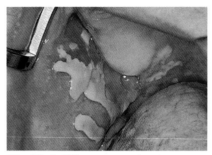

Fig 13-6 When requesting immuno-fluorescence to aid diagnosis of a vesiculo-bullous lesion the incisional biopsy must avoid the ulcerated region.

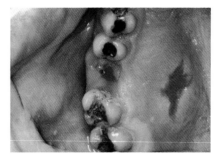

Fig 13-7 Palatal swellings should initially have incisional biopsies taken.

incisional biopsy should be first obtained so that a definite histopathological diagnosis can be made (Fig 13-7). Appropriate imaging of the underlying palatal bone should be carried out to check that there is no bony involvement. A computed tomography scan is the technique of choice, and thus referral to a specialist unit is recommended. If no bony involvement is seen, the lesion can be removed with supra-periosteal excision. Palatal mucosa granulates well in the resultant defect.

Curettings may also be sent for histopathological analysis. An example might be the soft tissue removed from the apex of a tooth at the time of apicectomy. This technique is also a form of biopsy.

Bony lesions in the mouth are invariably accessible via an intra-oral approach. A mucoperiosteal flap in the region of the lesion is reflected as for any other minor oral surgical procedure. The bone to be biopsied can be delineated with a fissure bur and the block removed using an osteotome.

Following the biopsy the site may be closed by approximating the wound edges to allow healing by primary intention. The use of elliptical incisions facilitates this. If primary closure is not possible, the defect can be packed with material such as Whitehead's varnish on ribbon gauze or a zinc oxide eugenol dressing held in place by sutures or added to a prosthesis.

The patient should be given a follow-up appointment for a date when the histopathological report will be available.

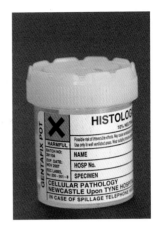

Fig 13-8 It is important that specimens sent for histological examination are transported in the appropriate medium. This container holds 10% buffered formalin.

Transfer of Specimens to the Laboratory

Once the specimen is removed it must be prepared for transport to the pathology laboratory. There are two types of specimen that can be presented to the laboratory. These are:

- fixed
- fresh.

Normally fixed specimens are sent from practice. The tissue is fixed by placing it into a vessel containing 10% neutral buffered formalin (Fig 13-8). This can be obtained from the local pathology laboratory. The volume of solution should be at least 10 times the volume of the specimen. The container should be labelled with the patient's details, which should include name and date of birth. If more than one specimen is removed it is recommended that they be placed in different containers identified by numbers.

A pathology request form should be completed. This should include the patient's details, including a relevant medical and drug history, date and site of biopsy, clinical appearance of the lesion and a provisional diagnosis. A drawing is useful and can help orientation by showing the position of any suture passed through the specimen.

If the specimen is to be sent by post to the laboratory appropriate packaging must be used. It is best to obtain information on this matter from the laboratory. However, as a minimum the container holding the specimen must be properly sealed and surrounded by material such as cotton wool, which

147

will absorb any spillage. This should then be placed in a sealed plastic bag and in a rigid container. The rigid container must be sealed and the outside labelled 'Pathological specimen – fragile – handle with care'.

A fresh specimen is needed if a vesiculobullous disorder is suspected. This is because immunofluorescence techniques will be used. Consultation with the laboratory to warn them of the imminent arrival of the sample and to ascertain precise requirements is always wise in these cases.

Aspiration Biopsy

A standard syringe and needle (e.g. a green 21 gauge needle) may be used to obtain fluid for analysis from suspected cysts or cyst-like lesions. Infection after this procedure is possible and the technique is therefore usually reserved for atypical lesions where neoplasia is suspected. In addition, in these circumstances it is usual to take a sample of soft tissue from the lesion wall.

Technique of fine needle aspiration biopsy

A 20ml syringe, 21 gauge needles, microscope slides and carriers, fixative spray and skin swabs are needed.
1. Air, apart from approximately 2ml, is expelled from the syringe and the needle attached.
2. The lump should be stabilised with the hand not holding the syringe, and the point of the needle should be inserted into the lump.
3. Apply suction to the syringe, maintain this and make several radial (1–5) passes within the substance of the lump.
4. Release suction and withdraw the needle from the lump. The cells are retained in the needle rather that transferred to the syringe.
5. Disconnect the needle and aspirate 10ml of air into the syringe.
6. Reconnect needle to syringe and expel aspirate onto a microscope slide.
7. A second slide is used to smear the specimen released onto the first slide.
8. Both fixed and air dried slides should be sent to the cytology laboratory for analysis.

Although the technique is simple in principle, it does need to be practised, and many acellular aspirates initially are not unusual. The presence of blood in an aspirate will not necessarily render it useless, but may cause an artefact on drying of the specimen.

If the lump being aspirated is malignant, seeding will not occur using FNAB, if the technique is performed as described above. It must be stressed again that if malignancy is suspected then urgent referral is essential and the biopsy should not be performed in general dental practice.

The Management of Intra-oral Calculi

A history of intermittent swelling of salivary glands may indicate the presence of a calculus in the draining duct. Other causes, such as a duct stricture, should also be borne in mind. Salivary calculi are most common in the ducts of the submandibular glands. On examination the calculus may be located by bimanual palpation of the floor of mouth (submandibular duct) or cheek (parotid duct). The obstruction may be sufficient to cause infection of the gland, and in these cases a bead of pus may be seen on initial 'milking' of saliva from the gland.

Radiography

Plain radiography is the investigation of choice in this context (Fig 13-9), but it should be remembered that not all calculi are radiopaque. In the case of the submandibular duct, the view of choice is a true occlusal radiograph of the floor of the mouth. Lateral views can sometimes be helpful, but bone is often superimposed.

For parotid duct calculi a dental film placed over the parotid duct orifice may demonstrate a calculus. Lateral views may again suffer from the superimposition of bone. An anteroposterior radiograph of the face when the patient has been asked to blow out the cheeks may be helpful.

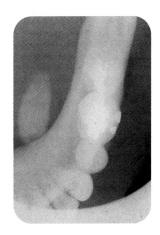

Fig 13-9 A lower occlusal radiograph showing a submandibular calculus.

Surgical Removal of Calculi via an Intra-oral Approach

Calculi can be removed by surgery or by retrieval using baskets attached to duct cannulation devices. As the latter are unlikely to be available in dental practice, only the surgical approach will be described.

Submandibular Duct

Removal of a calculus from the anterior part of the submandibular duct can be carried out under local anaesthesia. Acute infection may first be treated with antibiotics. Many surgeons place a temporary encircling suture around the duct posterior to the calculus (localised by bimanual palpation) to prevent it being pushed backwards into the gland. This should be tied fairly tightly. The duct is opened by a longitudinal incision over the calculus via an intra-oral approach (Fig 13-10a). Access may be improved by the assistant pushing up the floor of the mouth from the extra-oral side. The calculus is removed (Fig 13-10b) and either no suturing performed (Fig 13-10c) or the duct sutured open to prevent a subsequent stricture. If the calculus is situated too posterior in the duct (i.e. distal to the posterior border of the mylohyoid muscle), removal of the submandibular gland may be necessary to effect a cure. In such cases referral to a specialist oral and maxillofacial unit is required. If operating in the posterior part of the duct,

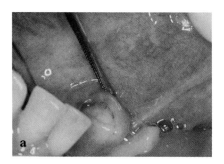

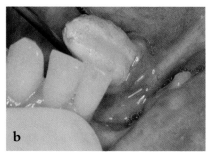

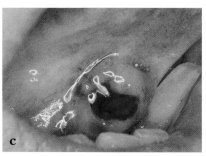

Fig 13-10 Removal of the submandibular calculus shown in Fig 13-9. (a) Incision over the calculus. (b) Removal of the calculus. (c) The incision is left patent to avoid stenosis of the duct.

care must be taken to identify and protect the lingual nerve, which crosses the duct in this region.

Parotid Duct

A similar technique to that described above may be performed for a calculus in the anterior parotid duct (including the posteriorly placed encircling suture) via an intra-oral approach under local anaesthesia. Calculi in this duct are present less frequently than in the submandibular duct. Calculi can be much more difficult to locate in this site, however. If the stone is located too far posteriorly, referral to a maxillofacial surgeon is needed, as a superficial parotidectomy will be required.

Conclusions

- Incisional and excisional biopsies are performed to confirm a diagnosis.
- Salivary calculi can be removed under local anaesthesia from an intra-oral approach.

Further Reading

Cawson RA, Odell EW. Essentials of Oral Pathology and Oral Medicine. Edinburgh: Churchill Livingstone 1998.

Kearns HP, McCartan BE, Lamey PJ. Patients' pain experience following oral mucosal biopsy under local anaesthesia. Br Dent J 2001;190:33-5.

Oliver RJ, Sloan P, Pemberton MN. Oral biopsies: methods and applications. Br Dent J 2004;196:329-33.

Chapter 14
Management of Complications and Emergencies

Aim

This chapter describes the complications and emergencies that can occur in the minor oral surgery patient.

Outcome

After reading this chapter you should understand the management of complications and emergencies in patients having minor oral surgery.

Introduction

Early recognition and prompt management of complications and emergencies distinguishes the experienced surgical practitioner from the novice. Perhaps of most significance, however, is the ability to identify potential difficulties at the time of patient assessment (see chapter 2).

Complications are usually the result of local surgical difficulties, whilst emergencies arise when generalised conditions threaten patient welfare.

Complications in Minor Oral Surgery

A complication may be defined as an unwanted event, rendering a surgical procedure more difficult, intricate or involved than previously expected. As in most clinical situations, forethought and preparation beforehand lessen their incidence.

It is helpful to divide complications into those arising during the immediate pre-operative phase, those occurring during surgery itself, and finally those that present post-operatively (Table 14-1).

Pre-Operative Problems

Limited access to the mouth creates obvious difficulties for minor oral surgery, and it may be better to postpone elective procedures when such conditions exist. Similarly, problems in achieving local anaesthesia or anxious

Table 14-1

Complications in minor oral surgery

PRE-OPERATIVE PROBLEMS

(A) Anatomical	– Trismus Small mouth Dental crowding Misplaced teeth
(B) Anaesthetic	– Difficulty or failure to achieve anaesthesia
(C) Patient cooperation	– Anxious patient Inadequate sedation

OPERATIVE DIFFICULTIES

(A) At surgical site	– Resistance to tooth extraction Tooth fracture Alveolar bone fracture Fracture of maxillary tuberosity Creation of oro-antral communication Haemorrhage Tooth/Root displacement Damage to instruments Failure to complete procedure
(B) At adjacent sites	– Extraction of wrong tooth Damage to adjacent teeth/restorations Damage to oro-facial soft tissues Inhaled or swallowed tooth/roots Fractured mandible TMJ trauma/dislocation

POST-OPERATIVE PROBLEMS

(A) Pain	– Tissue damage Acute alveolar osteitis (dry socket) Osteomyelitis TMJ injury
(B) Swelling	– Oedema Haematoma Infection

(C) Bleeding	– Upon completion of surgery Reactionary haemorrhage Secondary haemorrhage
(D) Trismus	– TMJ injury Muscular spasm Haematoma

patients with poor cooperation or unsuccessful sedation may require referral for hospital management. It is essential to take the medical history into consideration and adequately prepare the patient. Collapse of the patient during or immediately after giving a local anaesthetic is well recognised and should be managed promptly. Vasovagal syncope can be pre-empted in the nervous patient. It should be countered by ensuring that an adequate meal has been eaten prior to the appointment and by injecting the local anaesthetic with the patient in the supine position.

Operative Difficulties
Complications during extractions
These include:
- failure of pain control
- extraction of the wrong tooth
- fracture of the crown or root
- displaced tooth or root
- fracture of the bone
- damage to other structures
- broken instruments
- haemorrhage.

Failure of pain control
Pain during the extraction may be encountered and can be very disturbing both for the patient and the clinician. Collateral supply should be considered once the regional blockade of the sensory supply has been established. Periodontal ligament and intraosseous anaesthesia can be useful in some circumstances (Fig 14-1).

Extraction of the wrong tooth
This can occur if the clinician does not establish with the patient exactly

155

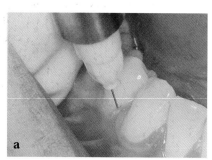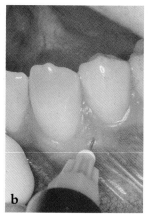

Fig 14-1 Periodontal ligament (a), and intraosseous (b) techniques are useful adjuncts when conventional approaches fail to provide complete anaesthesia.

which tooth is to be extracted. It is most likely to involve teeth of a similar morphology, such as premolars. The patient must be informed and reimplantation may be considered. However, the prognosis is not always favourable. In any case the planned extraction should be completed unless the tooth has been symptom-free.

Fracture of the crown or root
Whilst experienced clinicians often recognise and deal with abnormal resistance during tooth removal, crown or root fractures do occur at times due to pre-existing caries or restorations. It may also occur if the clinician relaxes the apical pressure on the tooth whilst moving the tooth buccally. In addition it may be the result of an abnormal root pattern. This should not be regarded as a major complication. The removal of the remainder of the tooth may require a surgical approach as described in Chapters 5 and 6. An assessment of the remaining fragment should be made concerning its size, proximity to important structures and the morbidity associated with its removal. Small apical fragments may be left in situ, as injudicious instrumentation may displace the remnant into the inferior alveolar canal or the maxillary sinus. If a decision is made to leave a root in situ (e.g. a third molar apex intimately related to the inferior alveolar nerve) the patient should be fully informed and an appropriate entry made in the case notes. The clinician should be prepared to proceed to a surgical approach if symptoms develop.

Displaced tooth or root

Displacement of teeth or roots may occur due to inappropriate elevation, and dental tissues may be forced into the maxillary antrum, infratemporal, pterygomaxillary or lingual spaces, the inferior alveolar nerve canal, pathological cavities or under mucoperiosteal flaps. Location and retrieval, if necessary aided by radiographic assessment, are necessary to prevent further complications. Difficulties may be encountered in the lower jaw if the fragment has been displaced lingually due to the presence of the lingual nerve. An upper third molar can be displaced upwards and backwards into the infratemporal fossa. This may make retrieval extremely difficult from an intra-oral approach. It may necessitate admission to hospital for an extra-oral approach. Thus this complication is best avoided. In order to prevent displacement of unerupted upper third molars into the infratemporal fossa, an instrument such as a Laster's retractor or a Howarth's periosteal elevator (Fig 14-2) should be placed behind the tooth when it is being elevated.

Care should be taken during the removal of the tooth from the mouth so that it is not inhaled or ingested. A dislodged tooth or root fragment that is accidentally swallowed and confirmed by radiography to be in the stomach or bowel may not need to be retrieved if it is seen to be passing through the alimentary tract. An inhaled foreign body definitely requires rigid bronchoscopy and removal to prevent lung collapse and infection. Immediate referral to hospital is essential if such a circumstance occurs or is suspected

Fracture of the bone

Fractures of the alveolar plate may occur during extraction of canine and molar teeth, whilst tuberosity fractures are often seen when lone-standing maxillary molars are removed, more commonly if they are unopposed. This

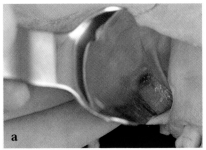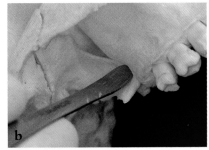

Fig 14-2 A Laster's retractor (a), or Howarth's periosteal elevator (b) is used to prevent posterior dislodgement of an upper third molar tooth.

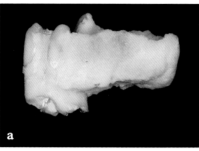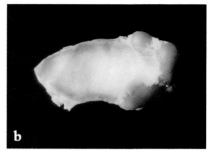

Fig 14-3 A fractured maxillary tuberosity. (a) Buccal view. (b) View from above showing the antral floor.

can lead to a large fragment of the posterior alveolus together with the associated teeth becoming mobile (Fig 14-3). The forceps extraction should be stopped and a surgical approach adopted to allow the tooth to be removed. Oro-antral communication (OAC) is a frequent occurrence in these circumstances, and careful closure to avoid the development of an oro-antral fistula (OAF) is essential (see Chapter 10). If the remaining teeth are mobile, they may require splinting until firm.

An OAC may also be created when maxillary molar teeth in close proximity to the antrum are extracted. Many small communications probably heal spontaneously, but immediate suture repair, instructions to avoid nose blowing and antibiotic prescription are advisable to encourage closure and prevent chronic OAF formation. Fistula excision and closure using buccal advancement (or more rarely palatal) flap repair are required to deal with large or long-standing fistulae (see Chapter 10).

Fracture of the basal bone is uncommon unless undue force is applied to a weakened jaw. Care should be taken to avoid this in elderly patients in whom gross resorption has occurred, or in the presence of pathology such as large dental cysts. When a fracture does occur, it is imperative that the surgeon recognises this and arranges further management without delay.

Damage to other structures
Adjacent teeth can be damaged inadvertently by the use of over large forceps or by inappropriate use of elevators. If it is likely that a filling or crown of an adjacent tooth will be dislodged due to the angulation of the tooth, the patient should be warned of this eventuality prior to the extraction.

With experience, damage to adjacent teeth or restorations should not occur, but unfortunately mishaps occasionally happen. It is important that the clinician is candid in discussing the events with the patient and is sympathetic and helpful in arranging any necessary additional treatment.

Soft tissues surrounding the tooth will be damaged to some extent during the extraction and may require suturing to reposition them satisfactorily. Damage to adjacent soft tissues such as the gingivae, lips, tongue, floor of mouth, related nerves (inferior alveolar, lingual or mental) and blood vessels must be recognised and repaired or managed appropriately.

The clinician or the patient may cause injury to the anaesthetised tissues of the mouth in the immediate post-operative period. Appropriate warnings concerning self-inflicted trauma should be given, particularly in the case of children who may have had no prior experience of local anaesthesia.

The temporomandibular joint (TMJ) can be damaged if the lower jaw is unsupported during the extraction. Patients with a TMJ problem can be helped during extractions by the use of a mouth prop on the opposite side. This allows them to clench their teeth and stabilise the joint.

Broken instruments
Instruments or burs occasionally fracture during surgery, and every effort must be made to retrieve retained metal fragments from the tissues.

Haemorrhage
Intra-operative haemorrhage can be alarming to both patient and surgeon. In addition, bleeding impairs access to the surgical field, which can prevent operative progress. Familiarity with local blood vessel anatomy and identification and ligation of vessels prophylactically can reduce the incidence of unexpected bleeding. Compression, haemostatic agents (e.g. oxidised cellulose), bone wax or suturing may be required to deal with established haemorrhage in dental practice (Fig 14-4). It is, of course, a basic principle that haemostasis is secured before completion of surgery.

Post-Operative Problems
Pain, swelling, bruising and trismus are, to some degree, inevitable sequelae of minor oral surgery, although careful tissue handling can reduce their severity. Extensive tissue damage predisposes to haematoma formation and post-operative infection. Damage to the inferior alveolar and lingual nerves was discussed in Chapter 6. The main post-operative problems are:

159

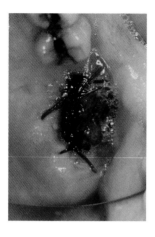

Fig 14-4 A haemostatic pack held in a socket with sutures to control haemorrhage.

- postextraction haemorrhage
- localised alveolar osteitis (dry socket)
- infection.

Postextraction haemorrhage
Medical screening pre-operatively should have identified patients at risk from systemic disorders. Those with conditions such as haemophilia should be referred to hospital for surgical treatment in coordination with the supervising haematologist. Thus most post-operative bleeding in dental practice is the result of local factors such as trauma, vascular lesions or infection. Haemostasis occurs within a few minutes of extraction in the normal patient but can be extended if the area is inflamed. Haemorrhage at some time after the extraction can occur when the vasoconstrictive effect of the local anaesthetic has worn off. This may be linked to the patient not following the postoperative instructions. Most haemorrhage can be controlled by sustained pressure. If this does not stop bleeding after 10 minutes then further measures are required. Sutures can be placed across dental sockets to exert pressure on the gingiva to arrest gingival bleeding. If the bleeding is from the depth of the socket, a haemostatic agent such as oxidised cellulose can be packed into the socket and held with a suture (Fig 14-4). Occasionally, it is necessary to raise a soft-tissue flap and ligate the vessel or apply bone wax directly to bleeding bone.

Reactionary haemorrhage occurs within 48 hours of operation due to a rise in local blood pressure, loss of vasoconstriction or opening up of previously constricted vessels. Secondary haemorrhage, which starts about seven days post-surgery, usually results from infection and blood clot destruction. The principles of managing post-operative bleeding are summarised in Table 14-2.

Localized alveolar osteitis (dry socket)
Painful acute alveolar osteitis (dry socket) may occur 24–72 hours following extractions, in particular after local anaesthetic removal of mandibular molar teeth in smokers. The condition arises due to dissolution of the blood clot, leading to an exposed bony socket. Pain relief, and local measures such as socket dressing are the mainstays of therapy. A number of materials are used as dressings including Whitehead's varnish on ribbon gauze, zinc oxide /eugenol packs or proprietary materials such as Alvogyl. This condition is described as extremely painful and may result in other teeth becoming sensitive. The temptation to extract further teeth should be resisted until the original socket is healing satisfactorily.

Table 14-2

Management of post-operative haemorrhage
Rapid review of operative and medical history
Assess patient's general condition and measure pulse and BP
Reassure patient and clean away excess blood
Examine mouth in good light with adequate suction
Locate the source of bleeding
Administer LA and apply pressure to wound
Suturing with or without packing of wound
Re-examine to ensure effective haemostasis
If still bleeding raise flap to ligate vessel or apply bone wax
Consider supportive treatment with analgesics, warmth, fluid replacement etc.
If bleeding persists, refer to maxillofacial unit for hospital admission and specialist management

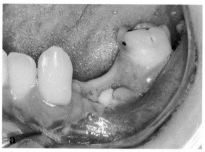
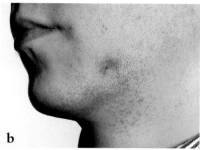

Fig 14-5 (a) An infected socket occurring in a patient suffering from diabetes. (b) The condition led to the production of an extraoral draining sinus.

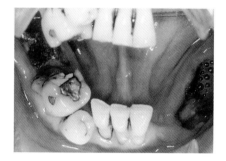

Fig 14-6 Necrotic bone and wound breakdown on both sides of the mandible following extractions in a patient with osteopetrosis.

Infection

Infection following extraction is quite rare given the excellent blood supply to the tissues. When infection occurs the clinician should be suspicious of the possibility of an underlying cause such as incipient diabetes (Fig 14-5a, b). The socket should be radiographed to exclude either a retained root or foreign body. A swab should be taken for microbiological culture and antibiotic sensitivity and appropriate antibiotics prescribed. A full blood count may reveal an underlying medical problem.

Osteomyelitis is a rare complication but can occur in immunocompromised patients, following radiotherapy to the mandible (osteoradionecrosis), or in patients with osteopetrosis (Fig 14-6).

Other serious infections are rare. If a post-operative infection is compromising the airway or if the floor of the mouth is raised due to an infective cause then early decompression is required. This should be performed under inpatient conditions, and immediate referral to a maxillofacial unit is needed.

Table 14-3 **Medical emergencies in clinical practice**

Medical emergency	
CARDIOVASCULAR	– Haemorrhage and hypovolaemia Chest Pain – Angina Myocardial infarction Stroke Acute cardiac failure Cardiac arrest
RESPIRATORY	– Asthma attack Respiratory obstruction Respiratory arrest
ENDOCRINE	– Hypoglycaemia in diabetics Corticosteroid insufficiency
ALLERGIES and DRUGS	– Anaphylaxis Drug reactions
NEUROLOGICAL	– Epileptic seizure Status epilepticus
PSYCHOLOGICAL	– Anxiety attack

Emergencies in Minor Oral Surgery

An emergency is an unexpected occurrence or situation demanding immediate action to prevent harm to the patient. Medical emergencies can occur suddenly, often with little warning. It is essential that all members of the surgical team appreciate the aetiology, diagnosis and effective management of these potentially life-threatening conditions.

Whilst up-to-date theoretical knowledge is important, all clinic staff should be involved with regular, practical exercises to rehearse how to deal with emergencies in the surgery.

Important medical conditions that can give rise to emergency situations are listed in Table 14-3. Careful pre-operative medical screening should identify patients at risk of developing acute chest pain, asthma or an epileptic

Table 14-4 **Management of collapse**

Cause	Clinical Features	Management
Faint	Dizziness, nausea, pallor, cold moist skin, slow weak pulse	Lay patient flat
Hypoglycaemia	Irritability, disorientation, drowsiness, warm moist skin, rapid full pulse	Oral glucose IM or SC glucagon (1mg) IV glucose
Corticosteroid Insufficiency	Pallor, rapid weak pulse, falling BP, loss of consciousness	Lay patient flat IV hydrocortisone (200mg) O_2
Anaphylaxis	Bronchospasm and laryngospasm, oedema, urticaria, itching, rapid weak pulse, falling BP, loss of consciousness	IM epinephrine (adrenaline) (0.5ml 1:1000) IV hydrocortisone (200mg) IV chlorpheniramine (10mg slowly) O_2
Stroke	Loss of consciousness, neurological deficit or paralysis	Maintain airway
Cardiac Arrest	Loss of consciousness, absent pulses, absent respiration, pallor or cyanosis	Summon assistance Cardiopulmonary resuscitation

seizure. Sensible use of regular medication by patients and the availability of drugs for emergency purposes are important precautionary measures.

The most significant (and frightening) mode of presentation of many emergencies is patient collapse. Collapse may be caused by faint (vaso-vagal attack or postural hypotension), hypoglycaemia, corticosteroid insufficiency, stroke, anaphylaxis or cardiac arrest. It is very important to recognise specific features associated with these conditions to ensure prompt diagnosis and management (Table 14-4).

Conclusions

- Complications can occur before, during and after surgical dentistry.
- Most complications are dealt with by local measures.
- Serious life-threatening complications require hospital admission.

Further Reading

Moore UJ (ed). Principles of Oral and Maxillofacial Surgery. 5th edn. Oxford: Blackwell Science, 2001.

Index

Quintessentials for General Dental Practitioners Series

in 50 volumes

Editor-in-Chief: Professor Nairn H F Wilson

General Dentistry, Editor: Nairn Wilson

Implantology in General Dental Practice	available
Culturally Sensitive Oral Healthcare	available
Dental Erosion	available
Managing Orofacial Pain in Practice	Autumn 2006
Dental Bleaching	Autumn 2006

Oral Surgery and Oral Medicine, Editor: John G Meechan

Practical Dental Local Anaesthesia	available
Practical Oral Medicine	available
Practical Conscious Sedation	available
Minor Oral Surgery in Dental Practice	available

Imaging, Editor: Keith Horner

Interpreting Dental Radiographs	available
Panoramic Radiology	available
Twenty-first Century Dental Imaging	Autumn 2006

Periodontology, Editor: Iain L C Chapple

Understanding Periodontal Diseases: Assessment and Diagnostic Procedures in Practice	available
Decision-Making for the Periodontal Team	available
Successful Periodontal Therapy – A Non-Surgical Approach	available
Periodontal Management of Children, Adolescents and Young Adults	available
Periodontal Medicine: A Window on the Body	available

Endodontics, Editor: John M Whitworth

Rational Root Canal Treatment in Practice	available
Managing Endodontic Failure in Practice	available
Preventing Pulpal Injury in Practice	Autumn 2006

Prosthodontics, Editor: P Finbarr Allen

Teeth for Life for Older Adults	available
Complete Dentures – from Planning to Problem Solving	available
Removable Partial Dentures	available
Fixed Prosthodontics in Dental Practice	available
Occlusion: A Theoretical and Team Approach	Autumn 2006

Operative Dentistry, Editor: Paul A Brunton

Decision-Making in Operative Dentistry	available
Aesthetic Dentistry	available
Communicating in Dental Practice	available
Indirect Restorations	Summer 2006
Choosing and Using Dental Materials	Autumn 2006

Paediatric Dentistry/Orthodontics, Editor: Marie Therese Hosey

Child Taming: How to Cope with Children in Dental Practice	available
Paediatric Cariology	available
Treatment Planning for the Developing Dentition	available
Managing Dental Trauma in Practice	available

General Dentistry and Practice Management, Editor: Raj Rattan

The Business of Dentistry	available
Risk Management	available
Quality Matters: From Clinical Care to Customer Service	available
Practice Management for the Dental Team	Autumn 2006
Dental Practice Design	Autumn 2006
Handling Complaint in Dental Practice	Autumn 2006

Dental Team, Editor: Mabel Slater

Team Players in Dentistry	Autumn 2006
Working with Dental Companies	Autumn 2006
Getting it Right: Legal and Ethical Requirements for the Dental Team	Autumn 2006
Bridging the Communication Gap	Autumn 2006
Clinical Governance	Autumn 2006

Quintessence Publishing Co. Ltd., London